T0206427

Cannabis Therapeutics
in HIV/AIDS

Cannabis Therapeutics in HIV/AIDS has been co-published simultaneously as *Journal of Cannabis Therapeutics*, Volume 1, Numbers 3/4 2001.

Cannabis Therapuetics in HIV/AIDS

Ethan Russo, MD
Editor

Cannabis Therapeutics in HIV/AIDS has been co-published simultaneously as *Journal of Cannabis Therapeutics*, Volume 1, Numbers 3/4 2001.

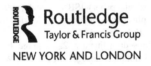
Routledge
Taylor & Francis Group
NEW YORK AND LONDON

Cannabis Therapeutics in HIV/AIDS has been co-published simultaneously as *Journal of Cannabis Therapeutics*, Volume 1, Numbers 3/4 2001.

First published 2001 by The Haworth Press, Inc.

This edition published 2010 by Routledge
605 Third Avenue, New York, NY 10017
4 Park Square, Milton Park, Abingdon, Oxon OX14 4RN

Routledge is an imprint of the Taylor & Francis Group, an informa business

ISBN 13: 978-0-7890-1699-7 (pbk)

Cover design by Marylouise E. Doyle

Photograph of Cannabis courtesy of GW Pharmaceuticals Ltd.

Library of Congress Cataloging-in-Publication Data

Cannabis therapeutics in HIV/AIDS/Ethan Russo, editor.
    p. ; cm.–(Journal of cannabis therapeutics; v. 1, no. 3/4)
    Includes bibliographical references and index.
    ISBN 0-7890-1698-2 (hard: alk. paper)–ISBN 0-7890-1699-0 (pbk.: alk. paper)
    1. AIDS (Disease)–Complications–Treatment. 2. Marijuana–Therapeutic use. 3. Cannabis–Therapeutic use. I. Russo, Ethan. II. Series.
    [DNLM: 1. HIV Infections–drug therapy. 2. Acquired Immunodeficiency Syndrome–drug therapy. 3. Cannabinoids–administration & dosage. 4. Cannabis. WC 503.2 C224 2001]
    RC606.6.C36 2001
    616.97'92061–dc21
                                                    2001051488

Cannabis Therapeutics in HIV/AIDS

CONTENTS

ABOUT THE EDITOR

Ethan Russo, MD, is a neurologist with Montana Neurobehavioral Specialists in Missoula. He is board certified in neurology with a special qualification in child neurology. In addition, Dr. Russo is Clinical Assistant Professor at the Department of Medicine at the University of Washington and Adjunct Associate Professor of Pharmacy at the University of Montana. He frequently lectures to undergraduate and graduate students in the fields of pharmacy, psychology, sports medicine, interpersonal communications, and physical therapy, among others. Dr. Russo has written numerous peer-reviewed articles on ethnobotany, herbal medicine, and cannabis, and has lectured internationally on these topics. He is also the author of the *Handbook of Psychotropic Herbs* (The Haworth Press, Inc.). Currently, Dr. Russo is actively engaged in bench research on the serotonin receptor activity of natural products, especially as it applies to migraine headaches.

Introduction:
Cannabis Therapeutics in HIV/AIDS,
Plus, a Modest Proposal

The *Journal of Cannabis Therapeutics: Studies in Endogenous, Herbal and Synthetic Cannabinoids* is pleased to present its first special issue, on the subject of *Cannabis Therapeutics in HIV/AIDS*. Certainly, with respect to therapeutic cannabis, HIV/AIDS sufferers are its most common consumers, and this is a topic most worthy of closer examination. Our current offering includes numerous articles pertinent to the issue, which will be supplemented by subsequent entries in future volumes.

The survey commences with a broad medical overview of the subject by Dr. Richard Bayer. This ably serves as a point of departure in its presentation of the pertinent topics of interest with respect to AIDS and its treatment.

Next, Clint Werner offers a distinct viewpoint, more of an "insider's view" on the twenty-year history of this affliction, and its interface with cannabis and the medical marijuana political movement.

Subsequently, we present two survey studies of clinical cannabis usage from different populations in California. Both confirm the assertion above that HIV/AIDS sufferers frequently turn to cannabis in attempts to treat their symptoms. The first is from Dr. Stephen Sidney, a physician and epidemiologist working for Kaiser Permanente, the state's largest HMO (Health Maintenance Organization). The second is from Valerie Corral, a clinical cannabis patient herself. Despite the fact that she is not from a professional background, her long-term study provides much useful information on the range of conditions, symptoms and results obtained with medical marijuana.

Dr. Guy Cabral provides us with a state-of-the-art review of immunological issues in cannabis usage. The picture is a cautionary one, but also one that pro-

[Haworth co-indexing entry note]: "Introduction: Cannabis Therapeutics in HIV/AIDS, Plus, a Modest Proposal." Russo, Ethan. Co-published simultaneously in *Journal of Cannabis Therapeutics* (The Haworth Integrative Healing Press, an imprint of The Haworth Press, Inc.) Vol. 1, No. 3/4, 2001, pp. 1-4; and: *Cannabis Therapeutics in HIV/AIDS* (ed: Ethan Russo) The Haworth Integrative Healing Press, an imprint of The Haworth Press, Inc., 2001, pp. 1-4. Single or multiple copies of this article are available for a fee from The Haworth Document Delivery Service [1-800-342-9678, 9:00 a.m. - 5:00 p.m. (EST). E-mail address: getinfo@haworthpressinc.com].

1

vides no blanket support or indictment of therapeutic cannabis with respect to immune effects. As always, more research is needed to ascertain all the medical implications inherent in this treatment modality.

Donald Tashkin provides another thorough review, this time of pulmonary issues with smoked cannabis that is of particular import to HIV-positive patients.

Early issues of *JCANT* have alluded to possible synergistic effects of cannabis components beyond THC. The following article by McPartland and Russo examines those "other players" in greater detail in an effort to elucidate the issue.

Moving into the area of harm reduction, Dr. Franjo Grotenhermen provides a clinician's interpretation of cannabis consumption issues, and a number of practical recommendations for patients and their doctors.

Dr. Dale Gieringer provides some of the first experimental data on the method of cannabis vaporization that portends to provide the same clinical benefits as smoking, but with markedly fewer health sequelae. This is a technology under intense scrutiny among clinical cannabis patients and advocates, but one hardly mentioned by the recent Institute of Medicine Report (Joy, Watson, and Benson 1999).

A research group from the University of Mississippi with lead author Susan Broom provides an experimental study examining another alternative cannabinoid delivery system, that of rectal suppositories containing THC-semisuccinate.

Rounding out the original articles, Drs. Brian Whittle, Geoffrey Guy and Philip Robson of GW Pharmaceuticals provide a glimpse of innovative research in the UK focusing on standardized sublingual whole-cannabis extracts, and aerosol preparations that many believe represent the future of standardized pharmaceutical cannabis delivery.

AIDS IN THE THIRD WORLD: A MODEST PROPOSAL

Since its discovery a mere two decades ago, acquired immune deficiency syndrome (AIDS) has quickly become one of the world's most challenging public health issues. Initial cases in the USA and Europe mostly affected homosexual males and intravenous drug abusers, making it easy for those in some quarters to relegate AIDS to some expression of heavenly revenge for immoral behavior. This introduced a noteworthy roadblock into funding for research (see Werner's article in this issue). When "innocent victims" such as transfusion recipients and babies with congenitally acquired infections appeared on the scene, public sentiments began to change. Soon enough, the disease proved to be a pandemic, and none was immune to its reach. It now affects 36 million people worldwide (Piot et al. 2001).

The current spread of AIDS is greatest in the Third World, with 60% of total cases in Africa, affecting an estimated 8% of the adult population (Thomas

2001). Transmission is primarily through heterosexual sex and vertical transmission. Asia seems to be the next nidus for its spread, which has recently been termed "explosive" (Kilmarx et al. 2000).

Treatment of AIDS remains extremely problematic, particularly in the Third World, due to the incredible expense of retroviral and newer protease-inhibitor drugs. These costs easily reach into the many thousands of dollars per patient per year.

Benefits of cannabis on appetite have long been known, including early citations by da Orta in India in his 1563 book (da Orta 1913), and Owen in the USA (Owen 1860). Sir William Dixon (1899), a noted pharmacologist, said of smoked cannabis (p. 1356), "It is not dangerous and its effects are never alarming, and I have come to regard it in this form as a useful and refreshing stimulant and food accessory, and one whose use does not lead to a habit which grows upon its votary."

The modern history of cannabis as an anti-anorexic and antiemetic is addressed in the current issue, along with two excellent reviews in the *JCANT* charter issue (Hollister 2001; Musty and Rossi 2001). Given the current support for this indication, and an overwhelming need for less expensive medicine to treat AIDS symptomatically until a cure is available, one might properly ask the question, "Why not cannabis?"

International law governing "illicit drugs" is contained within the United Nations Single Convention Treaty on Narcotics (United Nations 1961, available online at: *http://www.druglibrary.org/schaffer/legal/singconv.htm*).

Although international trade on cannabis is prohibited, existing provisions of the treaty allow for internal medical usage, or its abrogation in the event that the treaty contravenes a nation's constitution or its expression of human rights. That would certainly seem to be the case with AIDS. Increasingly, this treaty has proven counter-productive to the public health, and a key promotional factor in the highly wasteful and ineffectual international "War on Drugs." A modest proposal would call for its revocation, or at the very least, its amendment to allow for therapeutic cannabis usage as a stopgap effort in treatment of the worldwide AIDS epidemic.

Ethan Russo, MD

REFERENCES

da Orta, Garcia. 1913. *Colloquies on the simples and drugs of India*. London: Henry Sotheran.
Dixon, W.E. 1899. The pharmacology of *Cannabis indica*. *Brit Med J* 2:1354-1357.
Hollister, L.E. 2001. Marijuana (cannabis) as medicine. *J Cannabis Therap* 1(1):5-27.

Joy, J.E., S.J. Watson, and J.A. Benson, Jr. 1999. Marijuana and medicine: Assessing the science base. Washington, DC: Institute of Medicine.

Kilmarx, P.H., S. Supawitkul, M. Wankrairoj, W. Uthaivoravit, K. Limpakarnjanarat, S. Saisorn, and T.D. Mastro. 2000. Explosive spread and effective control of human immunodeficiency virus in northernmost Thailand: The epidemic in Chiang Rai province, 1988-99. *AIDS* 14(17):2731-2740.

Musty, R.E., and R. Rossi. 2001. Effects of smoked cannabis and oral delta-9-tetrahydrocannabinol on nausea and emesis after cancer chemotherapy: A review of state clinical trials. *J Cannabis Therap* 1(1):29-42.

Owen, P.H. 1860. A description of *Cannabis indica* with an account of experiments in its use. *NY Med Press* 3:280-283.

Piot, P., M. Bartos, P.D. Ghys, N. Walker, and B. Schwartlander. 2001. The global impact of HIV/AIDS. *Nature* 410 (6831):968-973.

Thomas, J.O. 2001. Acquired immunodeficiency syndrome-associated cancers in Sub-Saharan Africa. *Semin Oncol* 28 (2):198-206.

United Nations. 1961. Single Convention Treaty on Narcotics. New York.

Therapeutic Cannabis (Marijuana) as an Antiemetic and Appetite Stimulant in Persons with Acquired Immunodeficiency Syndrome (AIDS)

Richard E. Bayer

SUMMARY. Acquired immunodeficiency syndrome (AIDS) is a common cause of death among young adults in the USA. AIDS wasting syndrome is the most common clinical presentation of AIDS. Antiretroviral drug therapy has improved the prognosis of persons with AIDS, but also contributed side effects, particularly nausea and anorexia. Case reports demonstrate persons with AIDS use cannabis as medicine to control nausea, anorexia, and pain, while noting improved mood. Recent clinical research comparing smoked cannabis to oral dronabinol (synthetic THC or Marinol®) demonstrates no immune dysfunction in persons using cannabinoids and positive weight gain when cannabinoids are compared to placebo. Harm reduction research indicates that heating cannabis to temperatures well below combustion ("vaporization") yields active cannabinoids and a significant reduction or elimination of toxics (benzene, toluene, naphthalene, carbon monoxide, and tars) commonly found in smoked cannabis. More research is indicated but vaporizers appear to substantially reduce what is widely perceived as the leading health risk of cannabis, namely respiratory damage from smoking. In spite of a need for more rigorous scientifically controlled research, an increasing num-

---

Richard E. Bayer, MD, FACP, is board certified in internal medicine and a Fellow in the American College of Physicians–American Society of Internal Medicine. He lives in Portland, Oregon (E-mail: ricbayer@home.com).

[Haworth co-indexing entry note]: "Therapeutic Cannabis (Marijuana) as an Antiemetic and Appetite Stimulant in Persons with Acquired Immunodeficiency Syndrome (AIDS)." Bayer, Richard E. Co-published simultaneously in *Journal of Cannabis Therapeutics* (The Haworth Integrative Healing Press, an imprint of The Haworth Press, Inc.) Vol. 1, No. 3/4, 2001, pp. 5-16; and: *Cannabis Therapeutics in HIV/AIDS* (ed: Ethan Russo) The Haworth Integrative Healing Press, an imprint of The Haworth Press, Inc., 2001, pp. 5-16. Single or multiple copies of this article are available for a fee from The Haworth Document Delivery Service [1-800-342-9678, 9:00 a.m. - 5:00 p.m. (EST). E-mail address: getinfo@haworthpressinc.com].

ber of persons with AIDS are using cannabis to control nausea, increase appetite, promote weight gain, decrease pain, and improve mood. *[Article copies available for a fee from The Haworth Document Delivery Service: 1-800-342-9678. E-mail address: <getinfo@haworthpressinc.com> Website: <http://www.HaworthPress.com> © 2001 by The Haworth Press, Inc. All rights reserved.]*

KEYWORDS. Cannabis, marijuana, dronabinol, THC, Marinol®, AIDS, HIV, harm reduction, immunodeficiency, vaporization, vaporizer, wasting, anorexia, nausea, appetite, pain

AIDS IN THE UNITED STATES

The history of acquired immunodeficiency syndrome (AIDS) began in 1981 when the first five cases of AIDS were reported in the United States. Shortly thereafter, the disease was categorized as an epidemic. In 1984, the etiology of AIDS was found to be an RNA virus called human immunodeficiency virus (HIV). In 1985, a sensitive enzyme-linked immunosorbent assay (ELISA) was developed, and clinical testing for antibodies to HIV became possible.

By 1993, the United States Department of Health and Human Services (DHHS) listed AIDS as the most common cause of death among men aged 25 to 44 years (US DHHS 1995). By the end of 1998, the United States Centers for Disease Control and Prevention (CDC) estimated that nearly one million Americans had contracted HIV infection, one-third of whom were unaware of their affliction (CDC 1999).

By the end of 1999, a total of 733,374 cases of affected persons with AIDS (PWAs) had been reported to the CDC. Demographics revealed that 82% were men, and 18% were women. Only 1% were children less than 13 years of age. Forty-three percent of persons with AIDS were white, 37% black, 18% Hispanic, < 1% Asians and Pacific Islanders, and < 1% American Indians and Alaska Natives. Forty-seven percent of persons with AIDS were men who have sex with men, 25% were injection drug users, 10% were persons infected heterosexually, and 2% were persons infected through blood or blood products (CDC 1999).

HIV destroys CD4+ T lymphocytes, and laboratory measurements of "T Cells" indicate immune system damage. More recently, the technology of polymerase chain reaction has allowed the actual measurement of HIV RNA blood levels or "viral load" and this parameter is increasingly utilized clinically to help determine when to initiate and modify antiretroviral therapies (Saag et al. 1996).

The surveillance conditions for diagnosis of severe HIV disease or AIDS were originally defined by the CDC prior to the identification of HIV as the etiologic agent. Although surveillance criteria have changed over the years, the clinician should view HIV disease as a spectrum of illness that ranges from a primary infection, to the asymptomatic infected, to advanced disease or AIDS, which causes marked morbidity and mortality (Fauci et al. 2000).

For surveillance purposes, AIDS is defined by indicator diseases such as the AIDS wasting syndrome, *Pneumocystis carinii* pneumonia, or Kaposi's sarcoma in young adults. AIDS is identified in asymptomatic persons by laboratory tests such as CD4+ T lymphocyte counts of less than 200/mcl or a CD4+ T lymphocyte percent of total lymphocytes less than 14 (CDC 1992). Since 1992, scientists have estimated that about half the people with HIV develop AIDS within 10 years after infection, but this time varies greatly from person to person (CDC 2000).

AIDS wasting syndrome is an AIDS-defining condition, identified when a patient manifests involuntary weight loss of more than 10% associated with intermittent or constant fever and diarrhea or fatigue for more than 30 days in the absence of a non-HIV explanation. It is the initial AIDS-defining illness in 9% of patients with AIDS in the United States and thus is currently the leading initial clinical indication of AIDS (Fauci et al. 2000).

Standard antiretroviral treatments for HIV infection, such as zidovudine (AZT or ZVD) or lamivudine (3TC) can cause significant nausea. Treated patients often have difficulty maintaining baseline weight. In 1996, the United States Food and Drug Administration (FDA) approved the use of protease inhibitors, which when taken in combination with standard antiretroviral drugs can reduce viral load and markedly slow the progression of HIV/AIDS disease (CDC 1998).

A concern for many who take protease inhibitors is that the side effects can be more severe than those associated with standard antiretroviral drugs. As occurs with some persons receiving chemotherapy for cancer, patients with AIDS often find that the medicines they need to sustain their lives can produce side effects so intolerable that they become reluctant to maintain their treatments, or fail to take treatment regularly. This can be dangerous, for failure to maintain a regular medication schedule can lead to the development of treatment-resistant strains of HIV (CDC 2000).

CANNABINOIDS AS ANTIEMETIC AND APPETITE STIMULANT IN AIDS WASTING SYNDROME

Ethnobotany documents important medical uses of herbs, including cannabis (Russo 2000), but the first modern placebo-controlled trial that demonstrated efficacy of THC as an antiemetic in cancer chemotherapy was published in 1975 (Sallan et al. 1975). In the 1970's and 1980's, six American states engaged in clinical trials of smoked cannabis and oral THC to control nausea and emesis from cancer chemotherapy. These trials involved 748 persons who smoked cannabis and 345 patients who used oral THC capsules, and demonstrated that smoked marijuana can be a very successful treatment for nausea and vomiting following cancer chemotherapy (Musty and Rossi, 2001). A synergistic relationship of the combination of THC and the antiemetic prochloperazine was more effective than either drug alone, as suggested by past studies (Hollister 2001). These are important findings, because our most efficacious modern antiemetics, including well-tolerated serotonin antagonists like ondansetron (Zofran®), promise only about 80% efficacy (Zofran® package insert). In other words, in one out of every five treatment episodes, our best antiemetics demonstrate no efficacy. Although no studies have been done comparing ondansetron to cannabis, patients would be well served by studying efficacy of cannabinoids alone, or in combination with other antiemetics in persons who currently cannot control nausea and emesis with modern serotonin antagonists like ondansetron.

In 1992, the FDA approved the use of Marinol® (dronabinol or synthetic THC) for the treatment of AIDS wasting syndrome. Dronabinol has been shown to stimulate appetite, promote weight gain and improve mood in persons with AIDS in short term studies (Beal et al. 1995), while maintaining effectiveness and safety over during a longer (12 month) study (Beal et al. 1997). Marinol® is usually prescribed at a dose of 2.5 mg by mouth 2 to 3 times daily before meals to improve appetite (Roxane Labs 1999). Although the Drug Enforcement Administration (DEA) originally listed dronabinol as a Schedule II drug, it was recently moved to Schedule III, which may increase the likelihood of American physicians prescribing it.

While dronabinol is the only cannabinoid that physicians can legally prescribe in the USA, it remains extremely expensive (often $600 to $1200 US each month), has a slow onset of action because it can only be taken orally, and has a relatively high incidence of side effects (particularly dysphoria), so that many patients prefer herbal cannabis. As is the case in many cancer patients, people with AIDS frequently expressed a preference for smoked cannabis over dronabinol because it provides results with smaller doses and fewer undesirable side effects. In addition, some persons report better symptom control consuming cannabis rather than dronabinol, which may be related to the additional cannabinoids, such as cannabidiol, that are found in cannabis but not in dronabinol (Grinspoon et al. 1997).

Other agents used to treat AIDS wasting include anabolic steroid hormones such as the progesterone megestrol acetate (Megace®), tested alone and in combination with dronabinol (Wright et al. 1997), and androgenic steroids such as oral oxandrolone (Berger et al. 1996), or intramuscular testosterone enanthate (Grinspoon et al. 1998). More extreme options include human growth hormone, which can cost over $150 daily, and total parenteral nutrition, which is expensive, invasive, and medically risky (Krampf 1997). The above treatments have shown some successes, but all have drawbacks, and thus treatment must be individualized to meet each patient's needs.

For a more comprehensive discussion of cannabis as antiemetic and appetite stimulant, readers are referred to Leo Hollister's review, "Marijuana (Cannabis) as Medicine." in the charter issue of *Journal of Cannabis Therapeutics* (Hollister 2001). For a comprehensive clinical discussion of HIV disease, readers are referred to an internal medicine textbook such as *Harrison's Principles of Internal Medicine* (Fauci et al. 2000).

CASE REPORTS (THE PATIENTS' PERSPECTIVE)

There are many case reports from persons with AIDS who benefit from adjunctive use of cannabis to stimulate appetite, control pain, and improve quality of life (Zimmerman et al. 1998; Grinspoon et al. 1997; Krampf 1997).

Patient S.C. describes:

Within eight months, beginning in 1995, I was hospitalized three times for pneumonia and sinus infection. I'd been feeling pain and congestion in my chest, and then I began having trouble breathing. I was still taking AZT and they put me on antibiotics and prednisone for the pneumonia. It was so difficult for me to swallow the pills. Almost immediately after taking them, a violent nausea would set in. I couldn't eat or hold down any food. After a few weeks of this, my weight dropped down from 150 to 115 pounds.

I did what I could during that time to get relief. That's when I realized, almost coincidentally, that marijuana alleviated my nausea. When I took a few hits of marijuana, I felt better within five to fifteen minutes. It also gave me back my appetite. In a short time, I gained back almost all my weight, and I began feeling much healthier.

Just as importantly, my marijuana use would help me deal with the new drugs I'd soon be taking. They began combining AZT and another anti-viral drug, called 3TC, with a protease inhibitor called Crixivan®. I did notice a gradual improvement in my health, and my T-cell count started coming up. But the nausea I experienced was worse than anything I had felt with AZT alone. It was indescribable. It didn't seem like I had many choices though. I knew I needed these medicines to stay alive, even though the nausea they caused me was unbearable. So, I kept taking them, along with marijuana to control the nausea.

I have to tell you that I sincerely doubt I could have continued the treatment without marijuana. This is very important because, while there is no cure for AIDS, I believe these medications have actually reversed my disease and saved my life. What marijuana did, aside from making me feel better, was make these drugs tolerable for me.

Right now, my weight is up to 148 pounds. I take 16 pills a day, and I smoke marijuana before each meal to quell the nausea and stimulate my appetite. About one-half hour before I want to eat, I take three or four puffs. Usually, in about 20 minutes, I get the munchies and then I want to eat. It's still a struggle sometimes, but I'm healthier, stronger, and I enjoy living. (Zimmerman et al. 1998, pp. 48-49)

Patient G.S. summarizes his experience:

Even if I was not recovering [from AIDS], the relief would have been worth any bad effect the marijuana might have had. I could keep down food, and I could stop the aching. Also, I'm convinced that one of the worst things for my immune system was the stress my sickness caused me. Marijuana reduced my stress and it calmed my soul. It made me not worry so much about the difficult regimen of pills I had to take, or how I was going to get to the grocery store because I didn't think I'd be able to walk. Marijuana allowed me to accept the possibility that I might die, and yet, I believe, because I smoked marijuana, I lived. (Zimmerman et al. 1998, p. 53)

In the US, many persons with AIDS use cannabis daily to control nausea, increase appetite, decrease pain, and improve mood. Although case reports like those above are frequent, the federal drug bureaucracy has kept a virtual stranglehold on all clinical research into the safety and effectiveness of cannabis (Doblin 2000).

RECENT CLINICAL RESEARCH ON CANNABINOIDS, IMMUNITY, AND WEIGHT GAIN

After an Byzantine ordeal that lasted the better part of a decade (Doblin 2000), University of California-San Francisco (UCSF) researcher, Donald Abrams, MD, was finally able to do a study to compare the effectiveness of dronabinol (Marinol®) versus smoked cannabis versus placebo in persons with AIDS.

The results of Dr. Abrams's study, "Marijuana does not appear to alter viral loads of HIV patients taking protease inhibitors," were released July 13, 2000 by UCSF (Abrams 2000). The study found that patients with HIV infection taking protease inhibitors do not experience short-term (3 week) adverse virologic effects from using cannabinoids.

Of the 62 subjects who completed the inpatient study, values for 36 with undetectable HIV RNA levels remained unchanged through the trial. All 26 subjects with detectable HIV RNA levels experienced declines in those levels. Of those, the subjects who smoked cannabis or took oral dronabinol experienced slightly greater decreases in HIV RNA levels than did subjects who took the placebo, but there was no statistical difference between the three groups.

All three groups gained weight, thanks to regularly scheduled meals and available snacks. However, the subjects in the placebo arm gained an average of 1.30 kg, while those who took oral dronabinol gained an average of 3.18 kg, and those who smoked cannabis gained an average of 3.51 kg. These results should alleviate some concerns about the effects of THC as dronabinol and smoked herbal cannabis on immunity,

CANNABIS AND HARM REDUCTION STRATEGIES FOR PERSONS WITH AIDS

There is concern about risk of potential respiratory and lung infection in immunocompromised persons from smoking cannabis because underground market sources may be contaminated with bacteria or fungal spores. Some patients minimize this risk by cultivating their own cannabis, while others are careful to obtain cannabis only from trusted sources. Some persons heat the cannabis in a toaster oven for several minutes to reach the temperature used to pasteurize milk, 71°C (160°F), but keep the heat much lower than the 140°C to 190°C (284°F to 374°F), at which temperature the cannabinoids "vaporize" or "volatize" causing significant degradation of source material (Rosenthal et al. 1997; Gieringer 2001).

These are descriptions of some patients' strategies, but there are no controlled trials demonstrating increased risk for infection in cannabis-only smokers versus nonsmokers among persons with AIDS or any documented clinical benefit from attempting to sterilize the cannabis as described above.

Some patients try to reduce the risk of using contaminated cannabis by alternately smoking cannabis and cooking it in food. Some books on medical use of cannabis contain recipes (Rosenthal et al. 1997), or alternatively, patients may use a standard search engine on the Internet. Patients sometimes rely on smoked cannabis when the symptoms of nausea are so severe they are incapable of oral intake, but at other times, bake it into brownies or put in other food. In this way, the patient may get the immediate and effective relief that smoking provides, but when the need is less pressing, minimize the risk of smoking potentially contaminated cannabis through oral intake.

Oral ingestion of cannabis resolves the issues of smoking toxicity, but the harm-reduction issue is complicated by the United States' War on Drugs, which causes a "prohibition tariff" and increases cost by a factor of about 10. Estimates are that without cannabis prohibition, production costs would be $30 to $40 per ounce (Grinspoon 1997), but current street prices are about $300 to $400 per dry ounce for high-quality female flowers ("bud"). Eating cannabis, or making tea is expensive, and as for dronabinol, it has a slower onset of action. Oral THC also produces lower blood levels, and is less effective in controlling nausea when compared to smoked THC cigarettes (Chang 1979).

Inhalation of therapeutic drugs, such as treatment of asthma using metered dose inhalers, provides rapid onset of action and dose titration using the minimum effective dose (which minimizes drug side effects). Medical inhalation of cannabis provides similar advantages, but without vaporization, carries the risk of inhaling smoke. Therefore, one method to reduce harm from smoking is for patients to use only high medical quality cannabis, so there is a greater concentration of therapeutic cannabinoids per mass ingested.

Promising initial results from a study by California NORML (National Organization to Reform Marijuana Laws) and the Multidisciplinary Association for Psychedelic Studies (MAPS) demonstrate that patients may be able to protect themselves from harmful toxics in cannabis smoke by inhaling their medicine using an electric vaporizer (Gieringer 2001). Vaporization involves releasing cannabinoids by heating cannabis to temperature short of combustion, thereby eliminating or substantially reducing harmful toxics that are present in cannabis smoke. Gieringer reports traces of THC appearing at temperatures as low as 140°C (284°F) while significant amounts of benzene did not appear until 200°C (392°F) and combustion did not appear until around 230°C (446°F) or above. An aromatherapy device called the Volatizer® (www.volatizer.com) consisting of an electric heating element similar to an automobile cigarette lighter on a metal wand produces a temperature of 185°C (385°F) and is placed over the bowl of cannabis that sits inside the top of a 0.5 liter side-arm Erlenmeyer flask. Vapors are inhaled through a rubber tube connected to the side-arm of the flask. The Volatizer® reduced measured toxics (benzene, a known carcinogen, plus toluene and naphthalene), carbon monoxide, and tars when compared to combusting the cannabis by flame. More research is indicated, but vaporizers appear to substantially reduce what is widely perceived as the leading health hazard of cannabis, namely respiratory damage from smoking. Drawbacks to vaporization include cost (a complete Volatizer unit costs $250 US), and portability. Competing aromatherapy devices include using a thermocouple heat gun blown across the cannabis and collecting vapors in a chamber or bag (www.mystifier.com) or placing cannabis in one end of a small (pencil size) glass tube with the other end of the glass tube connected to a plastic tube for inhalation. The glass end with cannabis is then inserted in an "oven" that looks like an automobile oil filter and vapors are inhaled through the plastic tube (*www.vaportechco.com*). These two units are less expensive (about $150 US) than The Volatizer® but have not yet been laboratory tested. Other units are available, but until paraphernalia laws are relaxed and mass production of vaporizers is possible (e.g., using small batteries), vaporization remains an attractive but expensive harm reduction tool.

Simpler devices such as water pipes or "bongs" that combust the cannabis and draw the smoke through water before inhalation serve to cool the inhaled smoke, but there is no evidence that they reduce the ratio of tar and particulate matter to therapeutic cannabinoids (Gieringer 1994). There may be undiscovered health advantages from cooling the inhaled smoke or filtering out certain gases, but any advantage of a water pipe or bong over a joint to deliver smoked cannabis remains undocumented.

A medical records review of 452 daily cannabis smokers who never smoked tobacco showed a slight increase in clinic visits for colds, flu, and bronchitis over a 2 year period when compared to demographically similar group of non-smokers of either substance (Polen 1993). Although heavy cannabis smokers report "smokers' cough" (chronic bronchitis), there is no evidence that cannabis smokers who do not smoke tobacco will develop small airways disease, such as emphysema (Tashkin et al. 1997).

Patients should be advised to stop holding one's breath after inhaling smoke for this technique does not increase benefits from cannabis, but rather appears to increase risks of potentially dangerous deposits in the airways. Probably because the lifetime quantity of smoke consumed by cannabis smokers is typically far less than for tobacco smokers, there exists no clinical evidence that typical cannabis smokers have higher rates of respiratory cancer (Zimmer et al. 1997). However, recent reports from the United States (Zhang et al. 1999) and Europe (Carriot et al. 2000) suggest heavy cannabis smokers may increase risk of head and neck cancer with a strong dose-response pattern.

CONCLUSION

Many patients report that cannabis helped prolong their lives by enabling them to cope with some of the difficult symptoms and treatments associated with AIDS. In spite of a need for more rigorous scientifically controlled research, an increasing number of persons with AIDS are using cannabis because they find it controls nausea, increases appetite, promotes weight gain, decreases pain, and improves mood.

REFERENCES

Abrams, D. 2000. Marijuana does not appear to alter viral loads of HIV patients taking protease inhibitors. University of California at San Francisco press release. ©1999 Regents of the University of California. Alice Trinkl, News Director. Source: Jeff Sheehy (415) 597-8165. *http://www.ucsf.edu/pressrel/2000/07/071302.html*

Beal, J. R., L. Olson, J. Laubenstein, J. Morales, P. Bellman, B. Yangco, L. Lefkowitz, T. Plasse, and K. Shepard. 1995. Dronabinol as a treatment for anorexia associated with weight loss in patients with AIDS. *J Pain Sympt Manag* 10(2):89-97.

Beal, J.R., L. Olson, L. Lefkowitz, L. Laubenstein, P. Bellman, B. Yangco, J. Morales, R. Murphy, W. Powderly, T. Plasse, K. Mosdell, and K. Shepard. 1997. Long-term efficacy and safety of dronabinol for acquired immunodeficiency syndrome-associated anorexia. *J Pain Sympt Manag* 14(1):7-14.

Berger J., L. Pall, C. Hall, D. Simpson, P. Berry, and R. Dudley. 1996. Oxandrolone in AIDS-wasting myopathy. *AIDS* 10(14):1657-62.

Carriot, F. and Sasco, A. 2000. Cannabis and cancer. *Revue d'Épidémiologie et de Santé Publique* 48(5):473-83.

Centers for Disease Control and Prevention. 1992. 1993 revised classification system for HIV infection and expanded surveillance case definition for AIDS among adolescents and adults. *MMWR Morb Mortal Wkly Rep* 41(51):961-962. *http://www.cdc.gov/mmwr/preview/mmwrhtml/00018179.htm*

Centers for Disease Control and Prevention. 1999. CDC guidelines for national human immunodeficiency virus case surveillance, including monitoring for human immunodeficiency virus infection and acquired immunodeficiency syndrome. *MMWR Morb Mortal Wkly Rep* 48(RR-13). *http://www.cdc.gov/mmwr/PDF/RR/RR4813.pdf*

Centers for Disease Control and Prevention. National Center for HIV, STD, and TB Prevention, Divisions of HIV/AIDS Prevention. 1998. *Trends in the HIV and AIDS Epidemic, 1998. http://www. cdc.gov/hiv/stats/trends98.pdf*

Centers for Disease Control and Prevention. National Center for HIV, STD, and TB Prevention, Divisions of HIV/AIDS Prevention. 1999. *HIV/AIDS Surveillance Report* 11(2):5. *http://www.cdc.gov/hiv/stats/hasr1102.htm or www.cdc.gov/hiv/stats/hasr1102.pdf*

Centers for Disease Control and Prevention. National Center for HIV, STD, and TB Prevention, Divisions of HIV/AIDS Prevention. 2000. *Guidelines for the use of antiretroviral agents in HIV-infected adults and adolescents. http://www.cdc.gov/hiv/treatment.htm.*

Chang, A. 1979. Delta-9-tetrahydrocannabinol as an antiemetic in cancer patients receiving high-dose methotrexate. *Ann Intern Med* 91(6):819-824. *http://www.teleport.com/~omr/omr chang.html*

Doblin, R. 2000. Multidisciplinary Association for Psychedelic Studies (MAPS) website with additional references: *http://www.maps.org/mmj/mjabrams.html*

Fauci, A.S. and H.C. Lane. 2000. *Harrison's Principles of Internal Medicine. Harrison's Online Edition.* New York City: McGraw Hill, Inc.

Gieringer, D. 1994. The MAPS/California NORML marijuana waterpipe/vaporizer study. *MAPS Bull* 5(1):19-22. *http://www.maps.org/news-letters/v06n3/06359mj1.html*

Gieringer, D. 2001. *NORML-MAPS study shows vaporizers reduce toxins in marijuana smoke.* California NORML press release. ©2001 California NORML. (415) 563-5858. *http://www.canorml.org/research/vaporizerstudy1.html*

Grinspoon, L. and J. Bakalar. 1997. *Marihuana: The forbidden medicine.* New Haven, CT: Yale University Press.

Grinspoon, L. 1997. Testimony of Lester Grinspoon, M.D. before the Crime Subcommittee of the Judiciary Committee, U.S. House of Representatives on October 1, 1997. *http://www.rxmarihuana.com/testimony.htm*

Grinspoon S., C. Corcoran, H. Askari, D. Schoenfeld, L. Wolf, B. Burrows, M. Walsh, D. Hayden, K. Parlman, E. Anderson, N. Basgoz, and A. Klibanski. 1998. Effects of androgen administration in men with the AIDS wasting syndrome. A randomized, double-blind, placebo-controlled trial. *Ann Intern Med* 129(1):18-26.

Krampf, W. 1997. AIDS and the wasting syndrome. In M.L. Mathre (ed.), *Cannabis in medical practice: A legal, historical, and pharmacological overview of the therapeutic use of cannabis.* Jefferson, N.C: McFarland & Co.

Polen, M.R., S. Sidney, I. Tekawa, M. Sadler, and G. Friedman. 1993. Health care use by frequent marijuana smokers who do not smoke tobacco. *West J Med* 158(6): 596-601.

Rosenthal, E., D. Gieringer, and T. Mikuriya. 1997. *Marijuana medical use handbook: A guide to therapeutic use.* Oakland, CA: Quick American Archives.

Roxane Laboratories Package Insert with full prescribing information for Marinol® brand of dronabinol. Revised 1999. *http://hiv.roxane.com/prodinfo/marinol.html*

Russo, E. 2000. *Handbook of psychotropic herbs: A scientific analysis of herbal remedies for psychiatric conditions.* Binghamton, NY: The Haworth Press, Inc.

Saag M.S., M. Holodniy, D. Kuritzkes, et al. 1996. HIV viral load markers in clinical practice: recommendations of an International AIDS Society-USA Expert Panel. *Nature Med* 2:625-629.

Summary at *http://www.hivatis.org/viral.html*

Sallan, S.E., N.E. Zinberg and E. Frei. 1975. Antiemetic effect of delta-9-tetrahydrocannabinol in patients receiving cancer chemotherapy. *New Eng J Med* 293:795-797.

Tashkin, D., M. Simmons, D. Sherrill, and A. Coulson. 1997. Heavy habitual marijuana smoking does not cause an accelerated decline in FEV1 with age. *Am J Respir Crit Care Med* 155:141-148.

Timpone, J., D. Wright, N. Li, M. Egorin, M. Enama, J. Mayers, and G. Galetto. 1997. The safety and pharmacokinetics of single-agent and combination therapy with megestrol acetate and dronabinol for the treatment of HIV wasting syndrome. *AIDS Res Hum Retroviruses.* 13(4):305-315.

United States Department of Health and Human Services. 1995. National Center for Health Statistics. *Health United States 1995. http:// www.cdc.gov/nchs/data/hus_95. pdf.*

Zhang Z.F., H. Morgenstern, M. Spitz, D. Tashkin, G. Yu, J. Marshall, T. Hsu, and S. Schantz. 1999. Marijuana use and increased risk of squamous cell carcinoma of the head and neck. *Cancer Epidemiol Biomarkers Prevent* 8(12):1071-1078.

Zimmer, L. and J.P. Morgan. 1997. *Marijuana myths: Marijuana facts. A review of the scientific evidence.* New York and San Francisco. The Lindesmith Center.

Zimmerman B., R. Bayer, and N. Crumpacker. 1998. *Is marijuana the right medicine for you? A factual guide to medical uses of marijuana.* New Canaan, CT. Keats Publishing, Inc.

Zofran®, brand of ondansetron, package insert. 2000. Glaxo-Welcome Inc. *http://www.glaxowellcome.com/pi/zofran.pdf*

Medical Marijuana and the AIDS Crisis

Clinton A. Werner

SUMMARY. The sudden emergence of the AIDS epidemic and the initial lack of effective treatments politicized the patient population into demanding quicker development of and access to promising medications. When numerous AIDS patients demanded marijuana to treat the anorexia and wasting syndrome resulting from both illness and medications, the federal government's Public Health Service closed the only legal source of supply. The federal authorities' abdication of compassion and repression of research spawned a grassroots political movement that repudiated federal regulations. *[Article copies available for a fee from The Haworth Document Delivery Service: 1-800-342-9678. E-mail address: <getinfo@haworthpressinc.com> Website: <http://www.HaworthPress.com> © 2001 by The Haworth Press, Inc. All rights reserved.]*

KEYWORDS. Acquired Immune Deficiency Syndrome (AIDS), HIV, cannabis, marijuana, medical marijuana, delta-9-tetrahydrocannabinol, AIDS-wasting syndrome, azidothymidine (AZT), dronabinol

The AIDS epidemic was a crucial influence on the growth of support for the medical marijuana movement. When federal officials responded to an increasing number of requests for marijuana from a growing population of AIDS patients by closing the Compassionate Use Investigational New Drug (IND) Program that supplied the drug, a grassroots political movement was launched to protect patients from arrest. The numbers of HIV-positive patients, the po-

Clinton A. Werner, BA, MLS, is the author of a forthcoming book on the history of the medical marijuana movement.

[Haworth co-indexing entry note]: "Medical Marijuana and the AIDS Crisis." Werner, Clinton A. Co-published simultaneously in *Journal of Cannabis Therapeutics* (The Haworth Integrative Healing Press, an imprint of The Haworth Press, Inc.) Vol. 1, No. 3/4, 2001, pp. 17-33; and: *Cannabis Therapeutics in HIV/AIDS* (ed: Ethan Russo) The Haworth Integrative Healing Press, an imprint of The Haworth Press, Inc., 2001, pp. 17-33. Single or multiple copies of this article are available for a fee from The Haworth Document Delivery Service [1-800-342-9678, 9:00 a.m. - 5:00 p.m. (EST). E-mail address: getinfo@haworthpressinc.com].

litical prowess of AIDS activists and the frustrations of AIDS researchers had a profound effect on the revelation to the American public that, with regard to cannabis, the federal government favored prohibition over science and compassion.

The first hints of the coming epidemic appeared at the end of the 1970's and in early 1980 when doctors in New York City, San Francisco, and Los Angeles began to see rare and unusual illnesses appearing among young gay men. The June 5, 1981 edition of the Centers for Disease Control publication, *Morbidity and Mortality Weekly Report* printed the following notice (Center for Disease Control 1981, pp. 305-308): "In the period October 1980-May 1981, 5 young men, all active homosexuals, were treated for biopsy-confirmed *Pneumocystis carinii* pneumonia at three different hospitals in Los Angeles, CA" the report also noted that, "*Pneumocystis* pneumonia in the United States is almost exclusively limited to severely immunosuppressed patients." A second troubling *MMWR* alert soon followed that linked the development of a rare skin cancer, Kaposi's sarcoma, in gay men to the outbreaks of *Pneumocystis*. The following day news of the burgeoning epidemic was relayed to the general public by the *New York Times'* headline (Altman 1981), "Rare Cancer Seen in 41 Homosexuals."

The syndrome was quickly traced to a breakdown in the immune system, but the causative agent remained unknown. Panicky speculation attributed the dysfunction to everything from water fluoridation to marijuana contaminated with paraquat, a quaternary ammonium pesticide (Shilts 1987). Initially, the illness was referred to as Gay Related Immune Deficiency (GRID), but the appearance of GRID-related opportunistic infections among hemophiliacs, transfusion recipients and intravenous drug users confirmed that the infectious agent lacked specificity to sexual orientation, and it was renamed Acquired Immune Deficiency Syndrome (AIDS).

When AIDS emerged, researchers had no precedent or guide in dealing with this catastrophic collapse of their patients' immune systems. Without an identified causative agent, no treatments could be devised. Doctors were forced to pioneer treatment protocols, resorting to trial and error exploration of off label prescriptions for never-before-seen maladies such as opportunistic infections with *Toxoplasmosis gondii* and *Cryptosporidium parvum*. Dr. Donald Abrams, Assistant Director of the AIDS program at San Francisco General Hospital, recalled the early days of the epidemic (Bayer 2000, p. 70), "We didn't have anything to offer them. [They] died, and the deaths they died, I recall, were very terrible deaths; they were deformed and disfigured and wasted away, Kaposi's sarcoma lesions all over their bodies."

On April 23, 1984, the isolation of the human immunodeficiency virus (HIV) that causes AIDS was announced. Knowledge that the infectious agent is a retrovirus allowed investigators to target their search for effective treatments. Due to the lengthy and involved Food and Drug Administration (FDA) drug approval procedure, however, any promising drugs that were developed were years away from availability. In the meantime, thousands would die without treatments for HIV. There were also myriad problems getting research under way.

There were two possible paths to drug availability: through government-sponsored clinical trials, or by research funded by pharmaceutical corporations in hopes of finding marketable products. Neither the government nor the private sector was eager to develop treatments for AIDS patients. The pharmaceutical companies did not envision that the numbers of AIDS patients would yield enough profits to justify expending millions of dollars on drug research and development (Arno 1992). The advent of AIDS also coincided with the inception of the Ronald Reagan Presidential Administration, which was committed to making deep cuts in domestic spending. Many of these policies adversely affected the ability of the nation's public heath service to respond to the type of public health catastrophe that AIDS was and remains (Shilts 1987).

The fact that the primary population affected by AIDS was gay men had a profound effect on the Reagan Administration's response to the crisis. President Reagan had decried homosexuality and trumpeted the right wing moralism of the Christian Coalition, whose members had flocked to the polls to vote for the former actor. For the first four years of the epidemic, Reagan refused to even utter the word "AIDS." The Reagan-appointed director of the CDC, Dr. James O. Mason complained of having to discuss various forms sexual activity with total strangers (Shilts 1987). Whether the negligence was due to distaste or malice, NIH spending on AIDS was drastically inadequate. In 1982, NIH expenditure for research into Toxic Shock Syndrome equaled $36,100 per death, and that for Legionaire's disease was $34,841 per death. In fiscal 1982, the NIH expenditure per AIDS death was a mere $8,991 (Shilts 1987).

In 1983, the San Francisco Board of Supervisors allocated $2.1 million for AIDS programs. Coupled with the $1 million from the previous year, San Francisco's spending on AIDS "exceeded the funds released to the entire country by the NIH for extramural AIDS research" (Shilts 1987, p. 186). Half of the money was allotted to establish the world's first AIDS clinic at San Francisco's General Hospital, which opened in July 1983.

With no drugs specific to treat HIV, and few available to treat the opportunistic infections that accompanied the resultant immune failure, AIDS patients were desperate. A significant number of the early AIDS-infected population included men who had pioneered the gay rights movement. This was a politically sophisticated group that already had a large activist infrastructure in place when the epidemic appeared. Almost overnight, gay rights activists became AIDS activists, fighting not for equality but for existence. Pressure was brought to bear on the government through protests, marches and demonstrations. A powerful activist group emerged, AIDS Coalition to Unleash Power! (ACT UP) which spread across the country and later, across the globe.

Many members of the gay AIDS population were also well educated and traveled, and used these privileges to their advantage. AIDS patients began researching promising treatments, unapproved by the FDA, but available overseas or across borders, where drug approval and distribution is less stringently regulated. Patients traveled to Mexico and other countries to buy the illicit medications and smuggle them back to the USA, frequently employing techniques developed by marijuana traffickers. In 1987 the first "buyer's clubs" were established in San Francisco and New York City, where they functioned as underground pharmacies for smuggled treatments and alternative therapies such as vitamins and herbs (Arno 1992).

In order to find some effective drug against HIV, the National Cancer Institute (NCI) began soliciting the profit-minded pharmaceutical corporations for compounds for federally funded testing. In 1985 a compound, azidothymidine (AZT), showed some evidence of anti-HIV activity in the laboratory. Responding to pressure from activists and the public-at-large the FDA accelerated the rigorous 3-phase testing requirements and allowed AZT to be widely distributed upon initial evidence of clinical benefit (Arno 1992). For some patients, AZT was effective with manageable side effects. Others were plagued by intolerable headaches, loss of appetite, stomach upset, stomach pain and nausea or vomiting.

One of the primary killers of AIDS patients was a wasting syndrome that resulted from a number of illness-linked influences including oral thrush, anorexia and chronic diarrhea. Wasting is defined as the loss of more than 10% of baseline bodyweight (Bayer 2000). The fact that, for many, AZT further suppressed the appetite and frequently resulted in gastric distress was a dire situation for patients who were already wasting due to the primary disease (Richman et al.1987).

Although AZT was rushed to approval, it proved to be no magic bullet. At best it extended survival by months, slowing viral replication, but not eradicating it (Bayer 2000). It was a cruel irony that the side effects of the only approved antiviral drug for HIV mimicked and aggravated some of the most devastating symptoms of the illness. In order to be effective, the drug had to be taken on a regular schedule, at very frequent intervals through the day and night. This meant that the side effects never had an opportunity to subside. With constantly depressed appetites it was a challenge for PWA's (People with AIDS) on AZT to ingest enough calories to rebuild body mass. Patients affirmed that marijuana usage not only eased and abated the gastrointestinal distress from both illness and remedy, but induced a voracious hunger and a seemingly insatiable compulsion to eat, known as "the munchies." For many

AIDS patients, smoking or eating cannabis became a primary component of their unorthodox treatment arsenal.

In 1983, the first call from an AIDS patient extolling marijuana's benefits reached Robert Randall, founder of the Alliance for Cannabis Therapeutics (ACT). Randall, a glaucoma patient whose suit against federal agencies forced the establishment of the Compassionate Investigational New Drug program for marijuana, had devoted his life to promoting medical marijuana and working to make it a prescription drug. ACT was founded as a nonprofit organization to further this endeavor.

Randall's most successful campaign had been an effort to persuade state legislatures to pass legislation to protect medical marijuana users (primarily cancer and glaucoma patients) from arrest and prosecution. By 1983, 34 states had enacted legislation that made marijuana available though "research programs." Because of marijuana's classification as a Schedule I drug, with the presumption of no recognized medical benefits and a high abuse potential, it could only be distributed for research through the National Institute on Drug Abuse (NIDA). Thus, Randall and the other legal users were provided with marijuana through the IND research exemption, despite the fact that no data was collected. Similarly, the states could only obtain cannabis by enacting specific research programs.

Production of the cannabis for federally approved research was conducted at a 5-acre farm at the University of Mississippi under a contract with NIDA (Randall 1998). The growing demand for marijuana from states with established research programs vastly outpaced the cannabis farm's ability to supply the drug. California alone requested 1 million marijuana cigarettes from NIDA (Randall 1998). In order to meet the needs of the state programs a new production plan would have to be established with state-of-the-art production techniques. Rather than move in this direction, FDA officials turned to synthetic THC as a surrogate for whole cannabis.

A stable method for the delivery of synthesized delta-9-tetrahydrocannabinoid, or THC in sesame oil, was developed for research purposes in the 1970's (Rosenkrantz et al. 1972). Later research established that oral THC had antiemetic properties and was significantly better than a placebo in reducing vomiting caused by chemotherapeutic agents (Sallan, Zinberg and Frei 1975). Despite the clinical evidence of antiemetic activity for oral THC, the researchers suggested that smoking might be a preferable route of administration due to its more reliable absorption compared to gastrointestinal ingestion. Moreover, smoking provides greater opportunity for individual patient control by permitting the patient to regulate and maintain the "high" (Sallan, Zinberg and Frei 1975). Efforts to prepare an aerosol delivery system for THC failed due to (Olsen et al. 1976, p. 86), "excessive tack of the spray and hence poor transport to the lungs."

Despite the irregular absorption and unpredictable mental effects of oral THC, it was the only solution available to stem the push for medical marijuana from the states. On June 26, 1980, an FDA advisory panel rushed to approve, by just one vote, the distribution of synthetic THC pills to oncology patients through a NCI research program (Washington Post 1981, p. A1). Panel member Dr. Charles G. Moertel, director of clinical cancer research at the Mayo Clinic, criticized the action and decried (Washington Post 1981, p. A1), "the current political hysteria for the general release of THC. I wonder if perhaps the weight of this political pressure does not exceed the scientific evidence justifying release." Robert Randall protested the diversion from cannabis to THC, charging that (Washington Post 1981, p. A1), "federal agencies are using their control of the nation's legal marijuana supply to corrupt the intent of the state laws." Only six of 34 states with research laws managed to obtain actual marijuana cigarettes (Randall 1998; Musty and Rossi 2001). The rest of the states were provided with "marijuana capsules," which were actually oral THC pills.

The resulting studies with THC evidenced some anti-emetic activity and the studies with inhaled cannabis found it to be safe and effective against chemotherapy-induced nausea (Randall 1998). With evidence that THC was effective against nausea in hand, the FDA faced the challenge of bringing it to market as a prescription drug. NIDA's chief of research and technology, Robert Willette noted that (Tucker 1979, p. 33), "Since THC isn't patentable, it's going to take a lot of coercion by the government to get a pharmaceutical company to market THC."

The FDA found a distributor for the THC pills in Unimed, a small New Jersey-based company that had no prescription drugs on the market, just over-the-counter remedies, and was eager to expand. After clearing the FDA-approval procedures, THC was given the generic name, dronabinol and marketed as Marinol®. THC in the form of dronabinol was moved from a Schedule I to a Schedule II designation, alongside cocaine and morphine, which permitted distribution by prescription in June of 1985. Despite the fact that a synthesized and concentrated version of cannabis' most active compound was rescheduled, the source plant was not. With marijuana withheld, and synthetic THC available by prescription, the state medical marijuana research programs slipped into dormancy.

Along with leading the state movements for medical marijuana, Robert Randall, through ACT, was working for Congressional legislation to move marijuana into the Schedule II designation. Although a bill attracted a broad coalition of supporters, it never moved out of committee.

ACT was also a co-petitioner with NORML (National Organization for the Reform of Marijuana Laws) for public hearings into rescheduling marijuana. After years of litigation against the Drug Enforcement Administration (DEA) in pursuit of these hearings, they were held in front of the DEA's Administrative Law Judge, Francis Young in 1987 and 1988. Judge Young ruled that marijuana has "an acceptable medical use in treatment in the United States" and proclaimed that the Schedule I classification was "unreasonable, arbitrary, and capricious" (Young 1998, p. 68). On December 30, 1989, DEA Administrator Jack Lawn announced his rejection of Judge Young's directive to reschedule.

Between the time of Judge Young's decision and Administrator Lawn's rejection of it, Robert Randall received a call from an AIDS patient in Texas who had reversed his wasting condition with marijuana, but was now facing jail after being arrested for possession. The patient, Steve L. wanted to gain admission into the Compassionate IND Program. Steve's physician agreed to sponsor him and after months of wrangling with evasive agencies, he was approved. The shipment of NIDA joints reached Steve on January 25, 1990, just 18 days before he died (Randall 1991; Randall 1998). Randall wrote an obituary for Steve that ran in *High Times*, a magazine for marijuana users. At the end of the tribute was included the phone number for ACT's offices.

In Panama City, Florida, a young couple was in desperate trouble. Kenny and Barbra Jenks were slipping into the late stages of AIDS. They were impoverished, with few health care resources and had just been arrested by the local narcotics task force and charged with serious felony violations: manufacturing marijuana with intent to distribute. Whittled away to near-skeletal thinness by HIV, the Jenks had been urged to smoke marijuana at an AIDS-support group meeting. After the meeting, they had been slipped a joint, but being "straight arrows" were reluctant to try it. When they eventually did try the marijuana, they discovered the munchies and both began to regain some weight and vitality. The couple became regular users of small amounts of cannabis, but without reliable connections within the "drug culture" or black market they often went without their medicine. Rather than rely on chance, Kenny planted some seeds and had cultivated two short and scraggly plants when they were arrested.

Kenny Jenks, a hemophiliac, had contracted HIV through the clotting factor he took to prevent death from internal bleeding. Barbra, Kenny's high school sweetheart, had contracted the virus from him. When their trailer was raided and agents found the tubing and syringes used for infusing clotting factor, Kenny was accused of being a heroin addict who was growing cannabis to support his habit.

Out on bail, Kenny came across the issue of *High Times* with Steve L.'s obituary and called ACT. Upon hearing the Jenks' story, Randall endeavored to find them legal representation and improved medical care from an AIDS expert who was willing to sponsor their IND application (Randall 1991).

Randall quickly realized the Jenkses' public relations value for promoting the use of marijuana for AIDS patients. They were literally "Ken and Barbi wholesome": salt-of-the-earth, heterosexual, monogamous. They lacked the homosexual and IV-drug use baggage that right-wing opponents could seize on to distort the issue by discomforting Middle America.

In March of 1991, after Kenny and Barbra had endured the standard institutional delays and had their IND supplies in hand, they joined Randall for a press conference to announce the launch of a new ACT endeavor, Marijuana/Aids Research Service (MARS). The service of the organization was to provide AIDS patients and their doctors with a uniform template with which to apply to the FDA for a Compassionate Use IND. Randall explained (Randall 1998, pp. 359-360), "Prior to MARS, physicians who requested IND forms from the FDA could wait for weeks, even months for the forms. When the papers did arrive there was no explanation about how to complete the 31 questions . . . Physicians who once struggled for hours to answer arcane FDA questions, could sit with an AIDS patient, open a MARS packet, go through a checklist and put an application in the mail in under an hour." The MARS forms were promoted by the Jenks and distributed to AIDS organizations throughout the country.

The AIDS-patient population responded enthusiastically to MARS. Many gay men who comprised the bulk of the AIDS-infected population had a profound distrust of the culture of authority and had never believed the "reefer madness" propaganda. These were largely children of the "Woodstock Nation." They had smoked pot, dropped acid, demonstrated against the war in Vietnam, gleefully violated anti-sodomy laws, and marched for gay liberation. There was little or no stigma associated with cannabis use for these patients, and they were eager for any remedy that worked. Soon, dozens of Compassionate Use IND applications began arriving at the FDA.

In June of 1991, just 3 months after the launch of the MARS effort, the patients receiving Compassionate Use IND marijuana found that their monthly shipments of the drug had been interrupted. The reason for the withholding of the marijuana became clear on June 21 when Dr. James O. Mason, Chief of the US Public Health Service (PHS) and former director of the Centers for Disease Control (CDC), announced the closure of the Compassionate Use IND Program saying (Isikoff 1991, p. A14), "If it's perceived that the Public Health Service is going around giving marijuana to folks, there would be a perception that this stuff can't be so bad. It gives a bad signal . . . there's not a shred of evidence that smoking marijuana assists a person with AIDS." Mason, much as his good friend and booster, Utah Senator Orrin Hatch, was infused with a pious attitude of abstention and priggishness. As director of the CDC, confronting the expanding AIDS crisis, Mason (Shilts 1987, p. 399), "couldn't bring himself to utter the word 'gay' when he met a gay delegation during his first day on the job." In justifying his decision to close the program, Mason expressed concern that AIDS patients taking medical marijuana (Isikoff 1991, p. WH 19), "might be less likely to practice safe behavior."

In response to Mason's abrupt announcement, Robert Randall organized a media blitz that highlighted the patients who were IND cannabis recipients in order to illustrate the political and callous nature of the decision. The well-oiled AIDS activism machinery engaged over the medical marijuana issue and phone trees were activated. The PHS, FDA, DEA and the White House Office of National Drug Control Policy (ONDCP) were clogged with calls from desperate patients, confused loved ones and angry activists. The AIDS-activist group, ACT UP, led a medical marijuana protest in the form of a "die-in" which closed the headquarters of Health and Human Services (HHS). Randall recalled (Randall 1998, p. 380), "what the agencies did not anticipate was the onslaught of public anger . . . This aggressive telephonic battering had a profoundly corrosive effect on institutional morale."

Mason's sudden and unilateral decision for IND closure had cast the ONDCP in a particularly bad light and put the agency in an untenable situation. Less than two months prior to Mason's announcement, ONDCP Assistant Director Herb Kleeber had appeared on the NBC television network's *TODAY* show to caution the ill away from buying cannabis on the black market. Kleeber reassured patients that (Today 1991, p. 25), "no one's been turned down in the last two years. There are over 35 such IND's on the market currently and the waiting period usually is less than one month . . . They can get an exception from the FDA. That's the way to go rather than go out and break the law."

Mason's announcement made Kleeber and the ONDCP seem foolish at best and dishonest at worst. The White House drug policy staff seemed moved and disturbed by the desperation of the calls they received, and initiated a challenge to the Compassionate Use IND's termination. The resulting interagency battle forced the PHS to suspend the closure until the conflict could be resolved.

Mason had planned to completely end the program, forcing Randall, the Jenks and other IND recipients to switch to dronabinol, despite the absence of any clinical data showing it to be safe and effective for their diseases. The ONDCP staff, in contrast, felt that this approach was a duplicitous betrayal of trust. They wanted NIDA to continue providing marijuana to all of those approved to use it, including those who had never received their supplies. In a scolding letter to Mason, Ingrid A. C. Kolb, acting deputy director for demand reduction at the ONDCP, wrote (Ostrow 1992, p. A13), "For HHS to treat this matter as just another bureaucratic decision is unconscionable and, to me, shows an intolerable lack of compassion." With the conflict at a stalemate, the final decision was passed up to HHS Secretary Louis Sullivan. In March of 1992, Sullivan settled the issue with a compromise. The program would close, but the current recipients would receive marijuana for the rest of their lives or until cured. The approved but unsupplied patients, primarily people with

AIDS, were prescribed dronabinol in lieu of cannabis. For HHS, the fix was in and the issue was settled. But no one could explain how someone with nausea and vomiting was supposed to hold down a pill the size of a bath oil bead.

While Randall and the Jenks were promoting MARS, a grassroots medical marijuana movement was germinating in San Francisco. On the same day that Steve L. became the first AIDS patient to receive legal marijuana (Randall 1991), career cannabis dealer and gay activist Dennis Peron's home was raided by San Francisco narcotics officers. Peron operated a marijuana market in the predominantly gay Castro neighborhood and the bulk of his clients were HIV-positive. During the raid, Peron and his housemates, one of whom was in the late stages of AIDS, were physically and psychologically abused by being hogtied, threatened with weapons and taunted with homophobic and AIDS-phobic slurs. The only cannabis tied to Peron was a moderate amount of top-grade marijuana that he and his ill housemate, Jonathan smoked. Peron went free when he and Jonathan explained to the court that the marijuana was an effective medicine against wasting. Two weeks after the trial, Jonathan succumbed to his disease and Peron (1996) recalled, "I kept thinking about how I was going to get even and I kept thinking that every AIDS patient needs pot and that is where I got the idea for a club." Peron knew that if he could openly sell cannabis, with medical use as a justification and a shield, then he would be tormenting and humiliating the narcotics squad while helping the ill.

Peron's first step was to gather enough voters' signatures to qualify a "Hemp Medications" proposition for San Francisco's November ballot. The proposition (Prop P 1996, p. 1) advised "the state of California and the California Medical Association to restore hemp medicinal preparations to the list of available medicines in California."

Peron's timing was perfect. Coincidentally, Prop P qualified for the ballot just days before James Mason announced the Compassionate IND closure and benefited enormously from the resulting publicity and furor over the lack of cannabis for AIDS patients. San Francisco was playing David to the federal government's Goliath, and the local press loved it.

In November, Prop P passed with an impressive 78% of San Francisco's voters saying yes to medical marijuana. Peron celebrated the victory by opening a "cannabis buyer's club" based on the model of the Healing Alternatives Buyer's Club which had sold unapproved medicines to AIDS patients for years without harassment. And since jurors are taken from the voter registration rolls, Peron felt sure that 78% of any jury would vote to acquit him should trouble arise. Peron's clientele grew as word of his operation spread, with some patients and caregivers traveling in from out of state to buy a variety of cannabis products in a safe and clean environment.

When HHS Secretary Sullivan finalized the Compassionate Use IND's closure in early 1992, San Francisco County Supervisor Terence Hallinan initiated an effort inspired by Prop P, to protect local medical marijuana users from being arrested (Hallinan 1998).

At San Francisco General Hospital's Ward 86, the AIDS ward, an increasing number of patients were reporting benefits from using cannabis. The ward's "Volunteer of the Year" for two years running, "Brownie Mary" Rathbun, had earned her nickname by baking marijuana-laced brownies for her "kids with AIDS." In June, 70-year-old Brownie Mary was arrested in the process of baking a large batch of illegal confections. After admitting that she baked the brownies and drove them to San Francisco to give them to AIDS and cancer patients, Brownie Mary was arrested and charged with transporting marijuana, a felony. The arrest of a little old lady for baking marijuana brownies for AIDS patients was the ultimate human interest story and was beamed around the globe by CNN. Rathbun was defiant, vowing (San Francisco Examiner 1992, p. A6), "My kids need this and I'm ready to go to jail for my principles . . . I'm not going to cut any deals with them. If I go to jail, I go to jail."

Dr. Donald Abrams, Assistant Director of the AIDS Program at San Francisco General Hospital, was in Amsterdam attending the International AIDS Conference when he retired to his hotel room, turned on the television and saw the story of Volunteer of the Year, Brownie Mary's arrest.

Also watching as the Brownie Mary saga unfolded was Rick Doblin, founder of the Multidisciplinary Association for Psychedelic Studies (MAPS) which worked to facilitate clinical research into the therapeutic potential of Schedule I drugs. Seeing that Brownie Mary was a volunteer at the world's premier AIDS facility, Doblin sent a letter to the program suggesting that a clinical trial of cannabis as a treatment for AIDS wasting should be conducted at "Brownie Mary's institution" (Abrams 1995). The letter was forwarded to Dr. Donald Abrams who pioneered and directed community-based clinical trials for HIV through San Francisco General Hospital's Community Consortium.

Community-based clinical trials became a third avenue of drug approval, along with federally initiated trials and research by pharmaceutical companies. Doctors treating AIDS patients became researchers, providing the opportunity for the collection and assessment of clinical data. The first drug approved through community-based research was inhaled pentamadine for *Pneumocytis carinii*. Pentamadine had originally been given intravenously, but it was toxic to the kidneys and other organs. Inhaled, the drug was delivered directly to the lungs where it was needed, sparing the rest of the body from some degree of side effects. Therefore, the idea of an inhaled medicine was not anathema to Abrams.

Abrams had also witnessed patients and friends with AIDS using cannabis and seeming to benefit from it. He had seen no serious harm, as with alcohol or cigarettes, or any number of prescription drugs at his disposal. With so many patients using medical marijuana it seemed as though some data should be gathered in case there was some unknown harm. There were rampant assertions and assumptions that marijuana could further damage the immune system.

Abrams contacted Doblin, and collaboration began to design a protocol for a study of cannabis to treat the AIDS-wasting syndrome. Abrams and Doblin consulted with FDA researchers in designing the trial and ushered it through approval from hospital committees, state and university investigational review boards and the FDA. Efforts to move forward with the research, which would have compared control patients with patients taking dronabinol and patients smoking marijuana, hit a roadblock at NIDA. In order to conduct the trial, Abrams needed marijuana, which only NIDA could supply.

While Abrams and Doblin worked on obtaining cannabis for the study, the San Francisco Board of Supervisors passed a measure to designate medical marijuana use as the lowest police priority. They also declared "Brownie Mary Day" in San Francisco. Rathbun's charges were subsequently dropped in Sonoma County, and she became a local folk hero.

The passage of Prop P and the supporting resolution inspired other communities to take similar actions. As support for medical marijuana grew, so did its use. Dennis Peron moved his buyer's club from a studio apartment to a large former dance studio at one of the city's primary public transportation hubs and he invited the media in to see. Buyer's clubs began appearing in other locations, including New York, Seattle, and Key West.

More initiatives passed and the overwhelming public support for medical marijuana motivated California State legislators to pass a measure that would reclassify cannabis as a Schedule II drug available by prescription. Governor Pete Wilson vetoed the bill, appropriately noting that state law could not make a drug available by prescription.

At San Francisco General Hospital, Abrams was waiting for approval from NIDA of his request for a supply of cannabis for the AIDS-wasting study. For 9 months, Abrams queried NIDA officials about the status of his request and was stymied with assurances and apologies. In April of 1995, Alan Leshner, Ph.D., Director of NIDA informed Abrams that (Leshner 1995), "we cannot comply with your request." Leshner complained that (CNN 1996), "The study was flawed and I couldn't justify using our scarce resources . . . "

Abrams was infuriated and responded with a scathing letter. Abrams (1995) wrote:

> To receive the first communication from your office nine months after we sent the initial submission is offensive and insulting . . . The apparent absence of any possibility to discuss your concerns and to modify the protocol so that we may work together for the benefit of our patients is also unacceptable in my opinion . . . your concerns about the scientific

merit of the study have not been shared by a number of competent reviewers and investigators.

Abrams closed the letter with a blistering attack:

> Finally the "sincerity" with which you share my "hope that new treatments will be found swiftly" feels so hypocritical that it makes me cringe . . . You had an opportunity to do a service to the community of people living with AIDS. You and your Institute failed. In the words of the AIDS activist community: SHAME!

At this point in the history of the medical marijuana movement a confluence of political deception, scientific frustration and grassroots activism generated a dynamic synergy for reform. Activists used Leshner's rejection and Abrams' response as public relations weapons.

Shortly after NIDA's rejection of the AIDS study the California legislature passed a bill to exempt medical users from prosecution under state law. Governor Wilson also vetoed this bill, and passed the buck saying (San Francisco Chronicle 1995, p. A22), "the Clinton Administration said in August marijuana should not be used for any purpose," referring to Attorney General Janet Reno's refusal to call a moratorium on the arrest of medical users.

Dennis Peron's Cannabis Buyer's Club had grown to accommodate over 10,000 members and relocated to a vast 5-story building in the heart of downtown San Francisco (Peron 1996). It was from this location that a network of activists, patients and suppliers launched a ballot initiative to enact a law to protect medical marijuana users from state anti-marijuana laws. Simultaneously, Donald Abrams and his research team were retooling their clinical trial to obviate any claims from NIDA that it "lacks scientific merit."

California's ballot initiative process allows citizens to enact or repeal laws that legislators have failed to address satisfactorily. In the fall of 1995, California activists began gathering signatures to qualify a medical marijuana proposition for the 1996 election. The effort succeeded following an infusion of cash from a group of wealthy sympathizers and the campaign for Prop 215 began.

Alan Leshner was in a difficult position as director of NIDA. The legislation that established the Institute charged the agency to (NIDA 1972, p. 55), "develop and conduct comprehensive health education, training, research, and planning programs for the prevention and treatment of drug abuse and for the rehabilitation of drug abusers." By definition, NIDA was precluded from facilitating research into the benefits of illicit drugs. If Leshner had violated the mission statement of his Institute, he could face a spate of political assault aimed at embarrassing the Clinton Administration.

Rather than continue to take the heat of public displeasure, Leshner washed his hands of the responsibility and agreed to provide marijuana for any study that passed NIH peer review, a part of the funding process for government-sponsored research. Abrams and the THC study team believed that this would work to neutralize political considerations.

In August, just three months before Californians would vote on Prop 215, Abrams received a rejection notice from the NIH. When the peer review panel's comments arrived Abrams began to see how deeply the political reefer madness bias had penetrated. Abrams (1998, p. 166) wrote:

> Two of the three reviewers mentioned in their comments that they were unclear as to why the Consortium investigators would chose to conduct a trial with such a "toxic" substance. The final reviewer was concerned that if patients with AIDS wasting developed increased appetite following marijuana ingestion . . . that they may subsequently develop hyperlipidemia (high cholesterol and triglycerides) and atherosclerosis. The peer review panel seemed to have missed the point: the reason the substance was being studied was because it was being so widely used in the local community. The reviewers apparent lack of insight into the natural history of the HIV-wasting syndrome also was of concern to the once again defeated protocol team.

The rejection of the second proposed study of marijuana use by AIDS patients came at a time when federal mouthpieces, most notably Drug Czar Barry McCaffrey, were trying to make a strong case against Prop 215, and a similar but broader measure in Arizona, by claiming that (Russel 1996, p. A8), "There is not a shred of scientific evidence that shows that smoked marijuana is useful or needed. This is a cruel hoax that sounds more like something out of a Cheech and Chong show." The retired general's argument lacked authority, especially when countered with a world class researcher's complaint that (Kanigal 1996, p. C1), "The government is saying there are no scientific studies proving the medicinal benefits of marijuana, but they're also not letting studies be conducted."

On Election Day, 56 percent of California's voters said "yes" to medical marijuana. It was a decisive victory that was a powerful indictment of the government's unwillingness to deal honestly with the issue. Arizona's more sweeping measure, allowing for the medical use of all Schedule I drugs, passed with 65 percent of the vote. Rather than heeding the will of the voters and redirecting their efforts toward dealing with medical marijuana scientifically, federal authorities moved to squash the uprising. McCaffrey and other opponents insulted voters by saying that they were "asleep at the switch" or were duped by pro-drug millionaires. When this technique failed to illicit a *mea culpa* from the voting public, Attorney General Janet Reno, supported by HHS Secretary Shalala, McCaffrey, and Leshner, threatened that "U.S. Attorneys in both states will continue to review cases for prosecution and DEA officials will review cases for prosecution and DEA officials will review cases, as they have, to determine whether to revoke the registration of any physician who recommends or prescribes so-called Schedule I substances" and that doctors might face "further enforcement action" (CNN 1996). The grim and punitive nature of the press conference clearly illuminated the federal government's brutal indifference to the plight of medical marijuana users. The outcry against the announcement was swift, massive and seething. The public, physicians and their professional organizations were outraged. Editorials across the nation decried the action as an interference with the doctor-patient relationship. A group of San Francisco doctors and patients responded by filing a class action suit against Reno, McCaffrey and DEA Administrator Thomas Constantine for violating the First Amendment to the Constitution.

The eruption of anger was so profound that within a week McCaffrey had retreated from his "not a shred of evidence" soundbite and announced a $1 million review of scientific evidence on marijuana as medicine to be conducted by the National Academy of Science's Institute of Medicine. The NIH also rushed to conduct a 2-day workshop on medical marijuana that continued to invalidate the drug czar's "Cheech and Chong" rhetoric. Rick Doblin, who attended the workshop and was still promoting Abrams' efforts to conduct research assured him that (Doblin 1997), "NIDA, NIH, and the Clinton Administration will have a very difficult time convincing the press that the publicly announced new openness to research is more than a PR front and delay tactic if your next NIH grant gets rejected."

A month earlier, in January, Abrams had met with Leshner at NIDA and discussed the barriers to researching marijuana's benefits. Leshner emphasized to Abrams that the Institute was "the National Institute *on* Drug Abuse, not *for* Drug Abuse" (Abrams 1997). Consequently, Abrams and the marijuana team devised a study to assess the potential harm that marijuana or dronabinol might cause by interfering with the new AIDS drugs, protease inhibitors. The study also included examination of weight gain and other measures that could indicate if there was a therapeutic benefit of cannabis for the subjects.

This third submission by Abrams' team was given special attention in the reviewing process and was promptly approved. On May 12, 1998, the first patients were enrolled in the study and began a 21-day stay at San Francisco General Hospital, during which they were randomized to dronabinol, a dronabinol placebo, or 3.95% THC cannabis in the form of NIDA's cigarettes. Initial results of the study were presented at the XIII International AIDS Conference in South Africa. Early findings indicate that: "Cannabinoids, smoked or oral, do not adversely effect HIV RNA levels after 21 days exposure. Smoked marijuana and dronabinol lead to significant increases in caloric intake and weight" (Abrams 2000). The THC Study Team also suggested that, "Future trials should investigate the effectiveness of marijuana in: appetite stimulation/ weight gain, nausea, pain" (Abrams 2000). The long-sought research has made a significant contribution to validating the "anecdotal" claims of the tens of thousands of AIDS patients who have used cannabis medicinally. The publication of more detailed findings from the study is pending.

The government's "new openness to research" did not dissuade the public of the notion that federal agencies had placed politics before science. Eventually, medical marijuana initiatives similar to Prop 215 were passed by voters in Arizona, Oregon, Washington, Maine, Nevada, Alaska, and the District of Columbia. In Hawaii, the state legislatures defied federal policy by passing a medical marijuana bill.

When the $1 million IOM report was released in March of 1999, it cautiously affirmed the medical use of marijuana, suggesting that better methods of delivery than smoking be devised.

And although research is proceeding slowly, it is finally underway. NIDA relaxed its restrictions requiring NIH peer review for all medical marijuana research, but added a PHS review panel process before providing medical marijuana to researchers. Several studies are pending in California through a state-funded research program including investigations into marijuana for multiple sclerosis and peripheral neuropathy.

Currently, as evidenced by the success of state ballot propositions, the American general public has generally accepted the idea that cannabis is a safe and effective medicine. The experiences of desperate AIDS patients using medical marijuana helped to change the nation's perceptions of the drug from menace to medicine.

REFERENCES

Abrams, D.I. 1995. Letter: to Alan Leshner (National Institute on Drug Abuse).
Abrams, D.I. 1997. Personal communication.
Abrams, D.I. 1998. Medical marijuana: Tribulations and trials. *J Psychoact Drugs* 30(2):166.
Abrams, D.I. et al. 2000. *Short-Term Effects of Cannabinoids on HI-1 Viral Load.* Poster. XIII International AIDS Conference in Durban, South Africa.
Altman, L.K. 1981. Rare cancer seen in 41 homosexuals. *NY Times.* July 3: A20.
Arno, P.S. and K. L. Feiden. 1992. *Against the odds: The story of AIDS drug development, politics and profits.* New York: HarperCollins.
Center for Disease Control (CDC). 1981. *Morbid Mortal Weekly Rep* June 5:2.
Cable News Network (CNN). 1996. *Higher* Times.
CNN. 1996. Press conference: Barry McCaffrey et al. December 30.
Doblin, R. 1997. Fax: to Donald Abrams.
Hatfield, L.D. 1992. Brownie Mary arrested again. *San Francisco Examiner.* July 23:A6.
Hallinan, T. 1998. Personal communication.

Isikoff, M. 1991. HHS to phase out marijuana program. *Washington Post*: June 22:A14.

Isikoff, M. 1991. Compassionate marijuana use: Supplies for medical needs are in trouble. *Washington Post*: November 12: WH19.

Kanigal, R. 1996. Medical marijuana heads for Nov. 5 battlefield. *Oakland Tribune*: October 20: C1.

Leshner, A. (National Institute on Drug Abuse). 1995. Letter to Donald Abrams.

Olsen, J.L., J.W. Lodge, B.J. Shapiro and D.P. Tashkin. 1976. An inhalation aerosol of delta9-tetrahydrocannabinol. *J Pharmaceut Pharmacol* 28(1):86.

Ostrow, R. 1992. Delay in lifting pot ban to seriously ill is assailed. *L.A. Times*: January 31:A13.

Peron, Dennis. 1996. Personal communication.

Prop. P. 1996. 215-Medical Use of Marijuana. Initiative Statute. *California Ballot Pamphlet*: 58.

Public Law 92-255. 1972. *National Institute on Drug Abuse: National Council on Drug Abuse*: 55.

Randall, R.C..1980. Medical substitute for marijuana won't work. *Washington Post*: June 29:C1.

Randall, R.C. 1991. *Marijuana and AIDS: Pot, politics & PWAs in America*. Washington, DC: Galen Press.

Randall, R.C. and A.M. O'Leary. 1998. *Marijuana Rx: The patients' fight for medicinal pot*. New York: Thunder's Mouth Press.

Richman, D.D., M.A. Fischl, M.H. Grieco, M.S. Gottlieb, P.A. et al. 1987. The toxicity of azidothymidine (AZT) in the treatment of patients with AIDS and AIDS-related complex. *New Engl J Med* 37:92.

Rosenkrantz, H., G.R. Thompson, and M.C. Braude. 1972. Oral and parenteral formulations of marijuana constituents. *J Pharmaceut Sci* 61(7): 1106-1112.

Russel, S. 1996. U.S. Drug Czar visits Haight, denounces medical use of pot. *San Francisco Chronicle*. Aug. 16: A8.

Sallan, S.E., N.E. Zinberg, and E. Frei. 1975. Antiemetic effect of delta-9-tetrahydrocannabinol in patients receiving cancer chemotherapy. *New Engl J Med* 293(16): 795-797.

Tucker, L. 1979. Legal grass farm supplies government pot. *Amer Pharm* NS19(10): 33.

TODAY Show transcript. 1991. *NBC*: May 6: 25.

Young, F. 1988. In the matter of marihuana rescheduling petition, docket 86-22, opinion, recommended ruling, findings of fact, conclusions of law and decision of administrative law judge. September 6, 1988. Washington, DC: Drug Enforcement Administration.

Marijuana Use
in HIV-Positive and AIDS Patients:
Results of an Anonymous Mail Survey

Stephen Sidney

SUMMARY. While there is a great deal of anecdotal reporting regarding the medical use of marijuana in HIV-positive patients, there have been few systematic surveys performed. The prevalence of medical use of marijuana in HIV-positive and AIDS patients was assessed by an anonymous mail survey of 1970 attendees of HIV clinics in the San Francisco, Oakland, and South Sacramento medical centers of the Kaiser Permanente Medical Care Program (KPMCP) in California. Of 442 responders (22.4% response rate), 147 (33.3%) reported current use of marijuana for medical purposes. Among current users, the most common reasons for using cannabis were: to feel better mentally/reduce stress (79%), improve appetite/gain weight (67%) and decrease nausea (66%). Patterns of use were heterogeneous, with daily use of cannabis reported by 34% of current users. Nearly half of participants reported buyers' clubs as a source for obtaining cannabis, a finding of particular interest because of recent successful government efforts in closing down these clubs in California. In combination with other reported surveys, these data suggest that the use of marijuana for medical purposes is relatively common in HIV-positive and AIDS patients. *[Article copies available for a fee from The Haworth Document Delivery Service: 1-800-342-9678. E-mail address: <getinfo@haworthpressinc.com> Website: <http://www.HaworthPress. com> © 2001 by The Haworth Press, Inc. All rights reserved.]*

Stephen Sidney, MD, is affiliated with Kaiser Permanente Medical Care Program, Oakland, CA.

Address correspondence to: Dr. Sidney, Division of Research, 3505 Broadway, Oakland, CA 94611 (E-mail: sxs@dor.kaiser.org).

[Haworth co-indexing entry note]: "Marijuana Use in HIV-Positive and AIDS Patients: Results of an Anonymous Mail Survey." Sidney, Stephen. Co-published simultaneously in *Journal of Cannabis Therapeutics* (The Haworth Integrative Healing Press, an imprint of The Haworth Press, Inc.) Vol. 1, No. 3/4, 2001, pp. 35-41; and: *Cannabis Therapeutics in HIV/AIDS* (ed: Ethan Russo) The Haworth Integrative Healing Press, an imprint of The Haworth Press, Inc., 2001, pp. 35-41. Single or multiple copies of this article are available for a fee from The Haworth Document Delivery Service [1-800-342-9678, 9:00 a.m. - 5:00 p.m. (EST). E-mail address: getinfo@haworthpressinc.com].

KEYWORDS. Marijuana, cannabis, HIV, AIDS, epidemiology

INTRODUCTION

The medical use of marijuana has become a highly political issue in the United States, with several states having passed initiatives approving its use for this purpose in the face of prohibition of its use for any purpose by federal law. Cannabis has specifically been advocated as a therapeutic adjunct to ameliorate the nausea and loss of appetite commonly associated with the wasting syndrome in AIDS (Grinspoon and Bakalar 1993). Media reports estimated that in 1996 up to 11,000 San Francisco Bay Area residents with HIV infection or AIDS were utilizing cannabis buyers' clubs to obtain marijuana for medical use (Abrams 1998).

While there are many anecdotal reports regarding the use of marijuana in HIV-infected individuals, there are few data available on its prevalence in this population. In order to provide information regarding this important issue, we conducted an anonymous mail survey of HIV-infected patients in 3 medical centers of the Kaiser Permanente Medical Care Program in Northern California to determine the prevalence of medical marijuana use and information regarding reasons for use, frequency of use, and sources. We report here the findings of this survey.

METHODS

The study population was composed of the attendees of HIV clinics in the San Francisco, Oakland, and South Sacramento medical centers of the Kaiser Permanente Medical Care Program, a prepaid medical care program which provides medical care to over 25% of the population of the greater San Francisco Bay area. In order to comply with the legal and administrative concerns of Kaiser Permanente, we performed an anonymous survey, i.e., no identifying information was included on the questionnaire. The initial mailing was sent to San Francisco members in January 1998. Because of a low response rate to the initial mailing of a 6-page questionnaire (about 10%), we developed an abbreviated 4-page questionnaire containing key questions from the longer questionnaire and re-mailed it in a subsequent newsletter in May, 1998, thanking those who had responded and requesting questionnaire completion from those who had not. Oakland members also were mailed the 6-page questionnaire with a flyer from the clinic in May 1998, with a later mailing of the 4-page questionnaire in July 1998. South Sacramento members were sent only the 4-page questionnaire in August 1998. A total of 1,970 members were sent questionnaires (1,200 from San Francisco, 650 from Oakland, and 120 from

South Sacramento). A postpaid return envelope was provided for the question-naires.

The questionnaire was mostly composed of check-off responses (yes/no, or choices of categorical responses). Data from the questionnaire responses were entered and processed into a SAS data set. A section was provided at the end of the questionnaire for participants to voluntarily provide identification infor-mation and to indicate whether we could have permission to review their medi-cal records in the next year to determine if they had experienced medical complications from AIDS, and if they were interested in being notified about other research projects in the future. The questionnaire and survey procedures were approved by the Institutional Review Board of the Kaiser Foundation Re-search Institute.

RESULTS

A total of 458 questionnaires were returned. Voluntary self-identification was provided on 158 questionnaires from the San Francisco and Oakland cen-ters, of which 16 represented duplicate responses, i.e., responses to both the initial and follow-up mailing. For these 16 responders (including 10 current users of marijuana for medical purposes), the initial questionnaire was in-cluded and the follow-up questionnaire excluded. This left 442 questionnaires (22.4% response rate) for the analysis, of which 229 were from San Francisco, 166 from Oakland, and 47 from South Sacramento. AIDS diagnosis was re-ported by 50% of responders, with 48% of the responders HIV positive with-out AIDS (2% unknown). Current use of cannabis for HIV or AIDS was reported by 147 patients (33.3%; 147/442), with 276 patients (62.4%) report-ing that they did not employ it (19 [4.3%] unknown). The prevalence of current cannabis use was slightly higher for AIDS patients (35.7%) than for HIV-in-fected patients without AIDS (30.5%). The responses to several questions re-garding use in current users are shown in Table 1. The most commonly reported reason for using cannabis from the 5 specific reasons listed on the questionnaire was to feel better mentally/reduce stress (79%), followed by im-prove appetite/gain weight (67%) and decrease nausea (66%). One-half of the patients did not know whether their doctor approved of their use of marijuana; of the remainder, 85% (63 of 74) reported that their doctor approved of their use of marijuana. The predominant mode of ingestion of cannabis was smok-ing (95%). Daily use was reported by 34% of current users, with 7% reporting use of less than once per week. About one-half of users reported use of canna-bis once per day (49%), with 12% reporting use more than 3 times per day. The most common sources for obtaining cannabis were buying from a friend or someone you know (59%) and purchasing from a buyers' club (48%), with

TABLE 1. Responses of Current Users of Marijuana for Medical Purposes (N = 147) to Several Questions About Use

Question	Percent
Main reason(s) for using marijuana	
Feel better mentally	79
Improve appetite/gain weight	67
Decrease nausea	66
Decrease pain/discomfort	48
Decrease symptoms of other medications	39
Does your doctor approve of your use of marijuana?	
Yes	43
No	6
Don't know	50
Missing	1
Method(s) of marijuana ingestion used (current users)	
Smoking	95
Eating	20
Capsule	3
Days of marijuana use per week	
< 1	7
1-3	33
4-6	26
7	34
missing	1
Number of times marijuana used per day	
1	49
2-3	35
> 3	12
Missing	4
Current source(s) for obtaining marijuana	
Buy from a friend or someone you know	59
Buyers' club	48
Grow my own	16
Buy from someone you don't know	9
Other	1

16% reporting growing their own. The money currently spent per month for marijuana ranged from $0 to $500, with a median monthly cost of $80. Of the 55 current cannabis users who reported ever using Marinol®, nearly all (98% [54 of 55]) reported that cannabis provided better relief of their symptoms; the other reported identical relief from both marijuana and Marinol.

In order to estimate the potential effect of duplicate form completion by San Francisco and Oakland survey participants on the prevalence of current use, we applied the duplicate form completion (i.e., completion of both initial and follow-up questionnaires by the same participant) rate for self-identified survey participants and the prevalence of current marijuana users among responders who completed forms in duplicate to the "anonymous" questionnaires, i.e., questionnaires from participants who did not self-identify. Using these data, of the 253 "anonymous" questionnaires from San Francisco and Oakland, 26 would be duplicates (253 × 10.1%) including those of 16 current users (26 × 62.5%). This would result in a current use prevalence estimate of 31.5% (131/416), slightly lower that the 33.3% estimate noted earlier.

DISCUSSION

The current study is larger than any that have been published regarding medical marijuana use in HIV-positive and AIDS patients. While the interpretation of the results of this survey must be tempered by the low response rate, the 33% prevalence of medical marijuana use in HIV-positive patients is comparable to that found in the few other published surveys. Wesner (1996) reported that 36.9% of a sample of 123 patients in Honolulu with HIV-positive status or AIDS responding to a mailed questionnaire survey responded that they had used cannabis as therapy. One-quarter of 228 HIV sero-positive men in the Sydney Men and Sexual Health study reported therapeutic use of cannabis (Prestage, Kippax and Grulich 1996). Thirty-two percent (32%) of 72 patients at a clinic in Alabama reported current use of cannabis (Dansak 1997).

The data regarding frequency of use are of interest because they demonstrated a heterogeneous pattern. Daily users were in the minority, and 40% of the responders indicated use on 3 or fewer days per week. On days of use, about half the current users reported using cannabis only once per day. In a survey of 102 HIV-positive clients of buyers' clubs in San Francisco and Oakland, more frequent use was reported compared to the Kaiser Permanente survey, with 26% of patients reporting cannabis use 3 times per day compared with the 12% in the Kaiser Permanente survey reporting use of at least 3 times per days (Child, Mitchell and Abrams 1998). In the Alabama study, 17% (4 of 23) patients who were current cannabis users reported using in 6 to 10 times weekly with all others reporting less frequent use (Dansak 1997). The other surveys noted earlier did not provide data regarding the patterns of cannabis use in HIV-infected patients.

The data regarding the sources for obtaining cannabis are of particular interest because of the high prevalence of buyers' club use. Buyers' clubs achieved increased popularity in California after the passage of Proposition 215 in 1996 legalizing the medical use of marijuana, but most have been closed down subsequent to the passage of this measure as a result of federal enforcement efforts.

The major limitation of the study is the low response rate, resulting from the requirement for anonymous mailing and the resultant inability to directly contact non-responders in order to increase the response rate. Because of the anonymity requirements, we were also unable to perform comparisons of the characteristics of responders and non-responders. As noted in the results, it is likely that some individuals who did not identify themselves completed both the initial and follow-up questionnaire, but that the impact of this on the estimate of the prevalence of the current use of marijuana would be minimal.

In summary, a substantial proportion (33%) of the HIV-infected patients who responded to this survey reported the current use of cannabis as a medical treatment for a variety of symptoms. The patterns of use were heterogeneous. The results of this survey, in combination with other surveys that have been reported, suggest that the use of marijuana for medical purposes is relatively common in HIV-positive and AIDS patients.

AUTHOR NOTE

This research was funded by grant number R01 DA06609 from the National Institute on Drug Abuse. The author acknowledges Tracy Kendall and Diana Holt for overall coordination of the survey; Joseph Dimilia of the Oakland Medical Center, Maura Varley of the San Francisco Medical Center, and Margot Fermer of the South Sacramento Medical Center for coordination of the survey mailings; Michael Sorel for computer programming; and Carroll Child, Sylvia Thyssen, and Rick Doblin for assistance with development of the survey questionnaire.

REFERENCES

Abrams, D.I. 1998. Medical marijuana: Tribulations and trials. *J Psychoactive Drugs* 30(2):163-169.

Child, C., T.F. Mitchell, D.I. Abrams. 1998. Patterns of therapeutic marijuana use in two community-based cannabis buyers' cooperatives [Abstract #60569]. *Proceed-*

ings of the 12th World Conference on AIDS, Geneva, Switzerland, June, 1998, p. 1105.

Dansak, D.A. 1997. Medical use of recreational drugs by AIDS patients. *J Addict Dis* 16(3):25-30.

Grinspoon, L., and J.B. Bakalar. 1993. *Marijuana, the forbidden medicine*. New Haven, CT: Yale University Press.

Prestage, G., S. Kippax, and A. Grulich. 1996. Use of treatments and health-enhancement behaviours among IV-positive men in a cohort of homosexually-active men. [Abstract Th.D.5181] XI International Conference on AIDS, Vancouver, BC, Canada, July 1996.

Wesner, B. 1996. The medical marijuana issue among PWAs: Reports of therapeutic use and attitudes toward legal reform. *Working Paper No. 3*, Working Paper Series, Drug Research Unit, Social Science Research Institute, University of Hawaii at Minoa, June, 1996.

Differential Effects of Medical Marijuana Based on Strain and Route of Administration: A Three-Year Observational Study

Valerie Leveroni Corral

SUMMARY. Cannabis displays substantial effectiveness for a variety of medical symptoms. Seventy-seven patients took part in a study in California to assess the efficacy of organically grown *Cannabis sativa* and *indica* strains in treatment of various medical conditions via smoking or ingestion. HIV/AIDS was the most frequent condition reported, at 51%. Standardized rating forms provided 1892 records that were statistically analyzed. Results demonstrated that in the case of nausea and spasm, symptom expressions are definitely affected by various methods of cannabis administration. However, while *Cannabis indica* strains increased energy and appetite, it is useful to note that in treating nausea in HIV/AIDS and orthopedic diagnosis groups, *Cannabis sativa* and *C. indica* strains proved equivalent. *[Article copies available for a fee from The Haworth Document Delivery Service: 1-800-342-9678. E-mail address: <getinfo@haworthpressinc.com> Website: <http://www.HaworthPress.com> © 2001 by The Haworth Press, Inc. All rights reserved.]*

KEYWORDS. Cannabis, medical marijuana, *Cannabis sativa*, *Cannabis indica*, AIDS, HIV

Valerie Leveroni Corral is affiliated with Wo/Men's Alliance for Medical Marijuana, 309 Cedar Street #39, Santa Cruz, CA 95060, a collective of patients and caregivers, creating community, building hope, dissolving barriers, providing support and free medical marijuana since 1993. www.wamm.org (E-mail: info@wamm.org).

[Haworth co-indexing entry note]: "Differential Effects of Medical Marijuana Based on Strain and Route of Administration: A Three-Year Observational Study." Corral, Valerie Leveroni. Co-published simultaneously in *Journal of Cannabis Therapeutics* (The Haworth Integrative Healing Press, an imprint of The Haworth Press, Inc.) Vol. 1, No. 3/4, 2001, pp. 43-59; and: *Cannabis Therapeutics in HIV/AIDS* (ed: Ethan Russo) The Haworth Integrative Healing Press, an imprint of The Haworth Press, Inc., 2001, pp. 43-59. Single or multiple copies of this article are available for a fee from The Haworth Document Delivery Service [1-800-342-9678, 9:00 a.m. - 5:00 p.m. (EST). E-mail address: getinfo@haworthpressinc.com].

INTRODUCTION

Marijuana, whether *Cannabis sativa* or *Cannabis indica*, produces its medical and other effects by virtue of the concentration and balance of various active ingredients, especially the cannabinoids, which are unique to marijuana, but also including a wide range of terpenoids and flavonoids. Terpenoids are cannabis constituents that provide the characteristic strong odor of marijuana and hashish. Flavonoids are any of the flavone derivatives. The concentration and relative proportions of these ingredients depend on the plant's genetic structure and applied hybridization techniques, and as such, allow for a substantially varied outcome.

Little is known about how differences in constituent profiles translate into differences in therapeutic effectiveness. A range of effects has been ascribed to THC (tetrahydrocannabinol is the primary psychoactive component of marijuana) and CBD (cannabidiol, a compound related to THC) when administered in purified form. Studies are lacking on the differential clinical effects produced when varying "menus" of constituents are taken together.

Another factor bearing on the effects and the effectiveness of marijuana is the route of administration. Orally administered marijuana is absorbed more slowly than when delivered systemically (e.g., smoking, vaporizers). Moreover, the liver metabolizes orally ingested marijuana to produce a potent and long-acting cannabinoid (11-hydroxy-THC), which induces varied reactions in medical marijuana patients and is often not well tolerated. However, once more, there is little information available concerning the differential clinical effects of oral vs. smoked forms of marijuana.

A major obstacle to obtaining data concerning differential clinical effects is, of course, the illegality of medical marijuana use. Almost equally troublesome, however, is the widespread view that medical knowledge can be gained only through randomized controlled trials. It is becoming increasingly accepted that valid causal inferences can be, and frequently are drawn quite regularly in medicine without such studies. As such, observational studies are quite capable of generating useful information, provided due care is taken to keep careful track of the process. In this case, careful and consistent documentation would be required concerning: (1) which forms of marijuana are being taken and by what route, and (2) what outcome is experienced by patients.

The passage of Proposition 215 in California in 1996 legalized medical marijuana under state law, thus clearing some legal obstacles to research. Prior to the passage of Proposition 215, two or more cannabis buyers' clubs and our collective comprised of patients and caregivers were in operation. Several provider associations have been operating since that time despite harassment of some by law enforcement agencies.

Valerie Leveroni Corral founded the Wo/Men's Alliance for Medical Marijuana (WAMM) in 1993. WAMM is a collective of patients and caregivers attempting to create community, build hope, dissolve barriers, and provide support and medical marijuana at no cost to patient members who possess a signed and verified recommendation from a physician licensed to practice medicine in California. A genetically-monitored, organic, communal garden is tended by WAMM client/ participants under the direction of Mike Corral and Valerie A. Leveroni Corral.

A primary function in this community based educational system is the creation of a database of information regarding the treatment of different symptoms with distinct cannabis varieties. This is achieved through daily effectiveness surveys and statistical analysis (Appendix, Tables 17 and 18). Our present collection of data also includes measures of effectiveness of cannabis on autoimmune illnesses, such as systemic lupus erythematosis, as well the many other disorders, including muscular dystrophy, epilepsy, quadriplegia, paraplegia, Parkinson's disease, glaucoma, arthritis, fibromyalgia, depression and migraine. However, AIDS and HIV-related conditions are the most frequently represented among our clientele.

WAMM initiated a study in 1993 designed to address the question of differential clinical effects between *Cannabis sativa* and *C. indica* strains and hybrids, and also examining effects of inhaled and ingested routes of administration. This study is ongoing and now includes "blind" trials where the varieties used are not apparent to the participating patient. A statistician generated all presented analyses.

MATERIALS AND METHODS

The determination of the variety of cannabis was based on the country of origin of the seeds strains and physical characteristics of each plant variety. We assure the genetic purity through carefully controlled breeding techniques, substantiated by twenty-five years of experience in cultivation and propagation of cannabis. Personal interaction took place with patient use of cannabis in more than one hundred different terminal cases.

An assessment instrument form is provided weekly to participating patients (see Tables 17 and 18). The patient places a label from a weekly supply on the seven day form, denoting the variety and form of cannabis (inhaled or ingested), the number of "puffs" if inhaled medicine is used and the amount or weight employed. All participants were instructed in a specific method of inhaling. Patients were requested to use and denote dosages correlated to the relief of specific symptoms. Participants observed and rated symptoms before and after cannabis use to assess their severity. This was done upon rising from sleep in all cases except "insomnia" and prior to using any cannabis. Assessments were made weekly, at minimum, or as much as seven times per week, in order to assess effectiveness and of different strains upon different target symptoms.

Findings were derived from data gathered during the time period of June of 1993 into early 1997. Statistical analysis consisted of frequency analysis, paired T-tests of "before" and "after" scores on each measured symptom or condition, and a series of one-way ANOVAs on route of administration (either inhaled or ingested), cannabis strain, and diagnosis.

Because the therapeutic effects of cannabis are sometimes ascribed to its mood-altering effects, we also performed a correlation analysis of the change in mood score with other outcome variables.

Inhalation methods of cannabis consisted mostly of smoking, with some use of vaporization, although patient reports of effectiveness appear substantially lessened when this technique was employed. This could certainly depend on the quality of the vaporizer design.

Ingested forms of cannabis consisted of baked goods and "mother's milk" (a soymilk-based liquid), and a whole cannabis tincture made with pure grain alcohol with leaf or a combined blend of leaf and flowers. Strains of marijuana were *C. sativa* and *C. indica* and their hybrids. The morphological distinction between these strains was determined by experienced cannabis cultivators associated with WAMM, based on characteristic features of the two sub-species, varieties or strains.

These sub-species varied from week to week and included the following pure strains and hybrid strains: *C. sativa*, *C. indica*, as well as hybrids of both, being the identified female *C. sativa* × male *C. indica*, as well as the identified female *C. indica* × male *C. sativa*. We secured a method of analysis of the chemical content of test materials, although we believe that the findings may be subject to error. Results from a drug detection laboratory indicated that *C. sativa* measured: THC 23.7%, CBD < 0.1% and CBN < 0.1%. Results indicated that *C. indica* strains measured: THC 19.6%, CBD < 0.2% and CBN < 0.5%. Cannabis potency testing results by ElSohly Labs of the same sample of *C. sativa* after storage for eight months yielded a value of THC 17.6%.

RESULTS

Seventy-seven patients completed a total of 1892 forms (range 1-256, median 8) during the three-year study period. Of these, 43 were male (56 percent), 22 were female (29 percent) and 12 were not coded as to gender. The distribution of primary diagnoses is presented in Table 1.

Thirty-nine patients (51 percent) had HIV/AIDS; 14 (18 percent) had neurological diseases, and 7 (9 percent) had a principle diagnosis of cancer.

To avoid biasing results due to a large proportion of questionnaires being completed by relatively few patients, we standardized the analysis by reviewing a maximum of eight records per patient, the median number completed by study subjects. These records were randomly chosen. Accordingly, our analysis contained 432 records. Of these, 261 (61 percent) referred to *C. sativa* experiences; 65 (15 percent) were *C. indica*, while 105 (24 percent) were coded "other." Certain types of marijuana were donated or undeclared, we labeled these as "other" and included them in our findings. Ingested forms were also recorded (Table 4). Some entries were coded with missing information, entered as slang or incorrectly named; these were excluded.

Paired t-tests of before and after health status revealed that the following symptoms were relieved to a statistically significant extent by therapeutic cannabis (without regard to strain or route of administration): pain, energy, mood, nausea, appetite, and awareness. The remaining symptoms were not reliably relieved to the same extent. Table 5 and Table 6 show the scores on each variable. The magnitude of improvement was unrelated to clinical diagnosis, as determined in ANOVA (Table 10), with one exception: the degree of relief of nausea was greater in the HIV/AIDS group (4.54 units) than in the orthopedic group (1.58 units) to a statistically significant extent ($p = 0.04$).

We next performed ANOVA on the strain of marijuana ingested: *C. sativa* and *C. indica*. The mean change scores, "before" scores minus "after" scores for patients with each condition, were calculated. For the most part, some observed changes were unrelated to strain of marijuana. However, two symptoms, energy and appetite, were improved to a statistically greater extent by *C. indica* than by either *C. sativa* or "other."

C. indica produced a mean improvement in energy of 3.76 units (vs. 1.53 for *C. sativa* and 2.22 for "other") and a mean improvement in appetite by 5.22 units (vs. 3.41 for *C. sativa* and 4.32 for *C. indica*). These differences were significant at the 0.012 and 0.005 levels, respectively (Table 8).

ANOVA was then conducted using route of administration as the independent variable (Tables 6 and 7). For the most part, ingested and inhaled marijuana had similar magnitudes of effects. Only one symptom, spasm, showed preferential improvement using smoked over ingested marijuana ($p = .036$) (Table 6). Patients reporting "other" routes of administration had substantially less relief of nausea than patients inhaling or ingesting marijuana (Table 7).

It is reported that THC may reduce spasms associated with both neurological and non-neurological disorders (Hollister, 1986; British Medical Association Report, 1997). It is interesting to note that the non-psychoactive cannabinoid cannabidiol has been shown to exhibit anticonvulsant properties in certain animal studies. In the case of some patients it has been noted to reduce or prevent the onset of both spasms and seizures when used alone or as an adjunct medicine. It appears that there are receptor sites for cannabinoids that have beneficial effects on seizure activity.

Finally, analysis of the Pearson correlation coefficients between changes in mood scores and changes in other symptom scores revealed only a single statistically significant correlation, between mood and energy level (p = 0.035). Mood was not correlated with any other outcomes, including pain relief (p = 0.817) (Table 11).

DISCUSSION

We analyzed 432 records of therapeutic cannabis exposures, including information on strain (*C. sativa, C. indica*, or other), and route of administration (inhaled, ingested or other). The outcome variables consisted of scores to a series of questions on symptoms, completed by the patient both before and after administering cannabis medicines.

Results indicate that cannabis was uniformly effective in relieving symptoms across a wide range of diagnostic categories. No differences were observed in the extent to which symptoms were relieved based on diagnosis, except that patients with HIV/AIDS experienced more relief of nausea than patients with primary orthopedic diagnoses (Table 13).

On several occasions, terminally ill patients remarked upon a recurrent phenomenon, described as a "shift in consciousness" or "perception" allowing them to approach their impending death more "openly" or in a more "relaxed" manner. This is of particular interest, as each patient also reported a reduction in anxiety often associated with the dying process. Future studies will further examine measures anxiety in the cannabis patient population.

C. indica appeared to be superior to *C. sativa* and "other" in improving energy and appetite (Table 9). Otherwise, no differences in strain effects were observed. Route of administration had little effect on outcome in our series. Two symptoms, spasm (Table 6) and nausea (Table 7) showed preferential improvement with smoking as compared to ingestion. In no condition was the ingested route superior to smoking for symptom management.

Changes in mood were not correlated with changes in other outcomes except for a modest correlation with energy (Table 11). The finding that mood did not correlate with other outcomes casts doubt on the theory that therapeutic cannabis effects are related primarily to improvement in mood. Conversely, this may pertain with the notion suggested by some patients that mood is not necessarily correlated to the concept of "feeling better." In our findings, it appeared that mood was often independent of symptom expression. This result is interesting because it appears in written testimony by patients in their surveys that they believe changes in awareness or consciousness do affect overall healing. We plan to further examine the validity of these phenomena in future studies.

These findings support that few differences were noted by patients between *C. sativa* and *C. indica* strains and between ingestion vs. inhaled routes of administration. This is likely due to modest observed differences in cannabinoid content in the supplied strains. We hope that a reliable and accessible means of analysis will become available in the near future to further assess these hypotheses.

This study is limited by the lack of blinding. For this reason, in 1998 a revised protocol was instituted in which patients receive a one-week supply of therapeutic cannabis at a time without knowledge of particular variety provided. Patients continued completing forms on a weekly basis. This method of blinding is expected to provide a more rigorous test of any distinctions between *C. sativa* and *C. indica* strains. Results may have implications for subsequent crossbreeding of strains to maximize therapeutic effects.

This study is only a small first step in the attempt to develop improved cannabis medicines for affected patients. The most significant current limitation to this type of research is the absence of a convenient legal mechanism in the USA for analyzing cannabis samples for biochemical constituent content. Until this limitation is overcome, progress in this area will be slow at best.

On the other hand, we should not underestimate the value of clinical observation in judging cannabis strains and their differential clinical effects irrespective of chemical content. Thus, while the work we report here does not definitively address issues of chemical variability, we believe that our findings provide at the very least a good working hypothesis for use in future studies.

REFERENCES

Grotenhermen, Franjo. 2001. Practical hints. In *Cannabis and Cannabinoids: Pharmacology, toxicology and therapeutic potential,* edited by F. Grotenhermen and E. Russo. Binghamton, NY: The Haworth Press, Inc.

Iversen, Leslie L. 2000. *The science of marijuana.* Oxford ; New York: Oxford University Press.

McPartland, J. M., and P. L. Pruitt. 1999. Side effects of pharmaceuticals not elicited by comparable herbal medicines: the case of tetrahydrocannabinol and marijuana. *Altern Ther Health Med* 5 (4):57-62.

McPartland, John M., and Vito Mediavilla. 2001. Non-cannabinoids in cannabis. In *Cannabis and cannabinoids,* edited by F. Grotenhermen and E. B. Russo. Binghamton, NY: The Haworth Press, Inc.

APPENDIX

Purpose of the Project

- To determine if there are physical, mood and perception changes resulting from use of the test article.
- To determine if the method of delivery affects measures of effectiveness.
- To determine if different types of cannabis affect diagnoses and measures of effectiveness.
- To assess the correlation between changes in mood and other measures of effectiveness.

Summary of Population

N = 77
43 males (56%)
22 females (29%)
12 missing gender distinction (15%)

TABLE 1. Description of Population by Primary Diagnosis

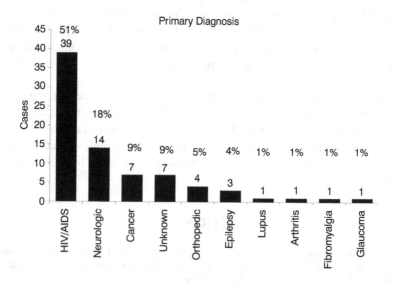

TABLE 2. Description of Patient Population by Secondary Diagnosis

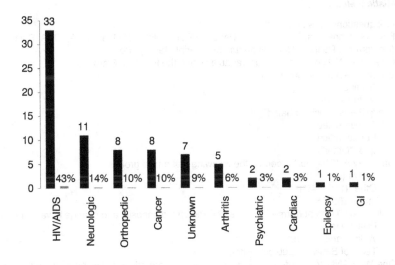

TABLE 3. Questionnaire Structure Measures of Effectiveness

Variable	None	Most	Desired Effect
Pain	1	10	Decrease
Energy	1	10	Increase
Mood	1	10	Increase
Nausea	1	10	Decrease
Appetite	1	10	Increase
Muscle Spasms	1	10	Decrease
Seizures	1	10	Decrease
Ocular	1	10	Decrease
Insomnia	1	10	Decrease
Awareness	1	10	Increase
Neuropathy	1	10	Decrease

Questionnaire Logistics

- 1892 Questionnaires Completed over 3 years
    Range of 1 to 256 questionnaires
    Average of 8 questionnaires/patient
    Analysis completed based on the average number of questionnaires completed (to normalize data for analysis)

TABLE 4

Statistical Methods

- 432 questionnaires analyzed
- Frequency analysis, Paired t-tests, Paired t-test correlations, One Way ANOVA, Post-Hoc (Bonferroni), Pearson Correlation and Multivariate tests performed
- One Way ANOVA conducted on variables using the following 3 groups
- Group 1–test article "ingested"
    Muffins
    Mothers milk
- Group 2–test article "inhaled"
    African Queen
    Purple Indica
- Group 3–"Other"
- One Way ANOVA performed on the following test article groups:
    Sativa (261–61%)
    Other (105–24%)
    Indica (65–5%)
- Multivariate Tests performed for type of Cannabis, diagnosis, and change in variable
    Pillai's Trace
    Wilks' Lambda, and
    Tests of Between-Subjects Effects
- One Way ANOVA, Bonferroni, Post-Hoc tests performed for definition of diagnosis and treatment effectiveness

All tests performed using SPSS (Statistical Program for Social Scientists) Version 9.0

TABLE 5

Question One

- Are there physical, mood and perception changes resulting from use of the test article?

Paired Samples t test

- Comparing means before and after
    95% confidence interval (2-tailed)

Variable	Before	After	Difference
Pain	6.98	3.26	-3.72 ± 3
Energy	4.12	6.04	1.92 ± 3
Mood	4.30	7.32	3.02 ± 4
Nausea	7.06	2.78	-4.28 ± 3
Appetite	3.02	6.96	3.94 ± 4
Awareness	5.73	6.97	1.24 ± 3

All are significant

TABLE 6

Question Two

- Does change in variable vary by method of treatment: ingested, inhaled or other?

Question Two–Means of Variable Changes by Mode of Consumption

	1	2	3	p
Pain	−3.75	−3.45	−3.67	0.274
Energy	2.05	1.14	1.18	0.630
Mood	2.98	2.54	3.81	0.840
Nausea	−4.39	−4.50	−2.22	0.934
Appetite	4.05	2.94	3.28	0.418
Spasm	−3.42	−3.95	−3.60	0.008*
Seizure	−0.14	N/A	−4.75	0.177
Ocular	−2.63	−2.54	−2.86	0.099
Insomnia	−3.88	−3.44	−4.28	0.036*
Awareness	1.31	−0.41	1.72	0.259

*Significant

ANOVA
Question Two

Examination of the mean change (One way Anova–95% confidence interval)
Significance was found for the following variables
Spasm   p = 0.008
Insomnia   p = 0.036

TABLE 7

Interpretation of ANOVA Method of Test Article Delivery

- Group 1 is different than group 3.
- Average group 1 (ingested) = −4.39.
- Average group 2 (inhaled) = −4.50.
- Average group 3 (other) = −2.20.
- There is greater improvement in nausea (0.36) with ingestables vs. "other."
- Ingestables and inhaled groups are not different.

TABLE 8

Question Three

- Are changes in variables related to the different types of cannabis and primary diagnoses?

Mean Change of Variables in Treatment Test Article Groups

	Other	Sativa	Indica	p
Pain	−3.49	−3.99	−2.93	0.078
Energy	2.22	1.53	3.06	0.012*
Mood	2.94	2.89	3.76	0.327
Nausea	−4.67	−4.19	−4.01	0.470
Appetite	4.32	3.41	5.22	0.005*
Spasm	−4.33	−3.53	−2.23	0.071
Seizure	−0.67	−2.12	0.50	0.316
Ocular	−3.27	−2.34	−3.00	0.646
Insomnia	−4.53	−3.82	−3.18	0.221
Awareness	1.75	0.96	1.24	0.173

One Way Anova–95% CI
*Significant

TABLE 9

Interpretation of ANOVA Method of Test Article Treatment Group

- The Indica Group is different than Sativa Group
    - Average Indica = 3.06
    - Average Sativa = 1.53
    - Average Other = 2.22
- There is greater improvement in energy (0.012) with Indica vs. Sativa and "Other."
- Sativa and Other treatment groups are not different.

Interpretation of ANOVA Treatment Group

- Indica was more effective to increase energy and appetite in any primary diagnosis group.
- Use of any test article was effective in treating Nausea in the Orthopedic and HIV/AIDS diagnosis group.

TABLE 10

Mean Change in Variable by Primary Diagnosis

	Ortho	Neuro	AIDS	Other	Cancer	p
Mood	4.36	4.05	2.87	1.33	2.64	0.001*
Pain	−4.93	−4.02	−3.31	−3.90	−3.27	0.011*
Energy	3.54	1.33	2.31	1.07	1.23	0.017*
Mood	4.36	4.05	2.86	1.33	2.64	0.094
Nausea	−1.58	−4.21	−4.54	−3.97	−4.18	0.015*
Appetite	4.57	3.50	4.44	3.08	3.00	0.010*
Spasm	−4.17	−4.05	−1.83	−3.29	−4.91	0.401
Seizures	NA	−1.86	−0.89	NA	NA	0.001**
Ocular	NA	−2.91	−2.00	−4.00	NA	0.334
Insomnia	−4.68	−4.66	−3.49	−2.93	−5.08	0.000*
Awareness	2.21	1.07	1.15	0.65	2.25	0.000*

One Way Anova 95% CI
*Significant
**Small sample size unable to correlate

TABLE 11

Interpretation of ANOVA Method for Primary Diagnostic Group

- The Orthopedic and Neurological group are different than the "Other" primary diagnostic group.
- There is greater improvement in Mood (p = 0.008) for the Orthopedic group vs. "Other."
- There is greater improvement in Mood (p = 0.001) for the Neurological group vs. "Other."

Average Orthopedic	4.36
Average Neurological	4.04
Average HIV/AIDS	2.87
Average "Other"	1.33
Average Cancer	2.64

- There is no difference between the AID/HIV and Cancer groups.

TABLE 12

Interpretation of ANOVA Method for Primary Diagnostic Group

- The Orthopedic group is different than the "Other" primary diagnostic group.
- There is greater improvement in Energy (p = 0.43) for the Orthopedic group than "Other."

Average Orthopedic	3.54
Average Neurological	1.33
Average HIV/AIDS	2.31
Average "Other"	1.07
Average Cancer	1.23

- There is no difference between the Neurological, AID/HIV, and Cancer groups.

TABLE 13

Interpretation of ANOVA Method for Primary Diagnostic Group

- The HIV/AIDS group is different than the Orthopedic primary diagnostic group.
- There is greater improvement in Nausea (p = 0.04) for the HIV/AIDS group than Orthopedic primary diagnostic group.

Average Orthopedic	−1.58
Average Neurological	−4.21
Average HIV/AIDS	−4.54
Average "Other"	−3.97
Average Cancer	−4.18

- There is no difference between the Neurological, Other, and Cancer groups.

TABLE 14

Interpretation of ANOVA Method for Primary Diagnostic Group

- There is improvement in Appetite (0.010) for all diagnostic groups.
- There is no difference in mean change for the Appetite variable for specific primary diagnostic groups.

Average Orthopedic	4.57
Average Neurological	3.50
Average HIV/AIDS	4.44
Average "Other"	3.08
Average Cancer	3.00

TABLE 15

Interpretation of ANOVA Method for Primary Diagnostic Group

- There is improvement in Insomnia (p = 0.000) for all diagnostic groups.
- There is no difference in mean change for the Insomnia variable for specific primary diagnostic groups.

Average Orthopedic	−4.68
Average Neurological	−4.66
Average HIV/AIDS	−3.49
Average "Other"	−2.93
Average Cancer	−5.08

TABLE 16

Interpretation of ANOVA Method for Primary Diagnostic Group

- There is improvement in Awareness (p = 0.000) for all diagnostic groups.
- There is no difference in mean change for Awareness specific to primary diagnostic groups.

Average Orthopedic	2.21
Average Neurological	1.07
Average HIV/AIDS	1.15
Average "Other"	0.65
Average Cancer	2.25

Correlation Analysis Question Four

- Is change in mood correlated to change in energy?
  p = .035*
- Is change in mood correlated to change in pain?
  p = .817
- Is change in mood correlated to change in nausea?
  p = .434
- Is change in mood correlated to change in insomnia?
  p = .647
- Is change in mood correlated to change in awareness?
  p = .073

*Significant

Conclusions

- There were observed changes in pain, energy, nausea, appetite, and awareness variables from the use of the test article.

TABLE 17

WAMM MEDICAL MARIJUANA EFFECTIVENESS SURVEY   *Wo/Men's Alliance for Medical Marijuana*

Please read the instructions on the other side of this page.

Name or ID: (Use your WAMM ID number if concerned about privacy. You may place the label from your medicine here.)	Gender	Age	Race	Diagnosis	Years since diagnosis

Weekly Medicine Allotment

Buds	Muffins	Milk	Brownies	Other

DAY:	WEDNESDAY		THURSDAY		FRIDAY		SATURDAY		SUNDAY		MONDAY		TUESDAY	
DATE:														
MEDICINE TYPE:														
DOSAGE UNIT:														
DOSAGE:														
CONDITIO\N	Before	After	Before	After	Before	After	Before	After	Before	After	Before	After	Before	After
Appeptite														
Awareness														
Consciousness														
Enegy														
Insomnia														
Libido														
Mood														
Nausea														
Neuropathy														
Ocular pressure														
Pain														
Seizures														
Spasms														

TABLE 18

Comments: (Use additional sheets of paper as needed. We are very interested in your comments.)

Instructions

Each day of the week, fill in the information BEFORE you take your medication for the first time in the day, and then again AFTER you take your medication for the first time of the day. Using a scale of 1 to 10, with **1 meaning WORST and 10 meaning BEST**, mark how you are feeling in the spaces provided. If the condition (symptom) improves, the number goes up.

Notice that the week begins on Wednesday in order to synchronize with our weekly meetings on Tuesdays.

If a condition does not apply to you, simply leave it blank.

Make sure to fill in at least one date.

Terminology

Appetite	Desire for food or drink	Medicine type	The code that appears on your medicine container or medicine name such as milk, muffins, brownies, buds.
Awareness		Mood	State or quality of feeling at a particular time. Prevailing emotional tone or general attitude
Best	Subjective experience of highest quality	Nausea	Sickness at the stomach, especially when accompanied by a loathing for food and an involuntary impulse to vomit.
Consciousness		Neuropathy	Symptoms of a diseased nervous system like tingly sensations.
Diagnosis	Name of disease such as cancer, HIV, glaucoma	Ocular pressure	Pressure within the eye
Dosage	Number of dosage units	Pain	Physical suffering or distress
Dosage unit	Name of dose, such as puffs, ounces, grams, bites, drops, fraction of weekly allotment (for example 1/7 means 1/7 of the weekly allotment.	Seizures	A sudden attack, as of epilepsy or some other disease
Energy	Capacity for vigorous activity	Spasms	Sudden, abnormal, involuntary muscular contraction
Gender	Male, female, transgendered	Worst	Subjective experience of lowest quality
Insomnia	Inability to sleep		
Libido	Sexual instinct or drive		

Developed by Rick Sinatra

Marijuana and Cannabinoids:
Effects on Infections, Immunity, and AIDS

Guy A. Cabral

SUMMARY. Marijuana and its major psychoactive component, delta-9-tetrahydrocannabinol (THC), alter resistance to bacterial, protozoan, and viral infections *in vivo* and *in vitro*. These alterations have been accompanied by modifications in functional components of the immune system. In addition, marijuana and THC, as well as other cannabinoids, have been reported to directly affect functional activities of lymphocytes, macrophages, natural killer cells, and other immunocytes. These include effects on cytokine production resulting in a shift in the balance of Th1 versus Th2 cytokines. Both receptor and non-receptor mediated modes of action have been proposed as causative of cannabinoid effects. Reports that marijuana and THC alter anti-microbial activity *in vivo* and *in vitro* indicate that its use presents a potential risk of decreased resistance to infections. However, few controlled longitudinal epidemiological and immunological studies have been undertaken to correlate the immunosuppressive effects of marijuana smoke or cannabinoids on the incidence of infections or disease in humans. *[Article copies available for a fee from The Haworth Document Delivery Service: 1-800-342-9678. E-mail address: <getinfo@haworthpressinc.com> Website: <http://www.HaworthPress. com> © 2001 by The Haworth Press, Inc. All rights reserved.]*

Guy A. Cabral, PhD, is affiliated with the Department of Microbiology & Immunology, Medical College of Virginia Campus of Virginia Commonwealth University, Richmond, VA 23298-0678.

Address correspondence to: Guy A. Cabral, PhD, Department of Microbiology & Immunology, Virginia Commonwealth University, Medical College of Virginia Campus, 1101 East Marshall Street, Richmond, VA 23298-0678 (E-mail: gacabral@hsc. vcu.edu).

[Haworth co-indexing entry note]: "Marijuana and Cannabinoids: Effects on Infections, Immunity, and AIDS." Cabral, Guy A. Co-published simultaneously in *Journal of Cannabis Therapeutics* (The Haworth Integrative Healing Press, an imprint of The Haworth Press, Inc.) Vol. 1, No. 3/4, 2001, pp. 61-85; and: *Cannabis Therapeutics in HIV/AIDS* (ed: Ethan Russo) The Haworth Integrative Healing Press, an imprint of The Haworth Press, Inc., 2001, pp. 61-85. Single or multiple copies of this article are available for a fee from The Haworth Document Delivery Service [1-800-342-9678, 9:00 a.m. - 5:00 p.m. (EST). E-mail address: getinfo@haworthpressinc.com].

KEYWORDS. AIDS, HIV, cannabinoid receptors, cannabinoids, delta-9-tetrahydrocannabinol, immunity, infections, marijuana, THC

INTRODUCTION

Marijuana, *Cannabis sativa*, is a highly complex substance that contains in excess of 400 chemical entities. Among these is a group of compounds classified as cannabinoids of which some of its 66 or more members exert a variety of effects on cells of the immune system. The cannabinoid that has been linked to the majority of the immunosuppressive effects attributable to marijuana is delta-9-tetrahydrocannabinol (THC), its major psychoactive component. Studies using *in vitro* and *in vivo* experimental models have indicated that marijuana or THC affects cell-mediated immunity (Klykken et al. 1977; Smith et al. 1978), humoral immunity (Mishkin and Cabral 1985), and cellular defenses against infectious agents (reviewed in: Cabral and Dove Pettit 1998; Friedman and Klein 1999). Compromised resistance in mice, rats, and guinea pigs to infection with amebae (Burnette-Curley et al. 1993), herpes simplex virus (Morahan et al. 1979; Mishkin and Cabral 1985; Cabral et al. 1986a; Cabral et al. 1986b; Fischer-Stenger et al. 1992), Friend Leukemia virus (Specter et al. 1991), *Listeria monocytogenes* (Morahan et al. 1979), *Staphylococcus aureus* (Baldwin 1997), *Treponema pallidum*, and *Legionella pneumophila* (Klein et al., 1993; Klein et al. 1994; Newton et al. 1994) has been reported. Although there are numerous reports relating to the deleterious effects of THC, this cannabinoid also has been reported to have therapeutic potential (Munson and Fehr 1983; Dewey 1986). It exhibits anti-nociceptive properties, has the ability to reduce intraocular pressure and bronchial constriction, and acts as an anti-convulsant and anti-emetic agent. Major advances have been made in the pharmacology and molecular biology of cannabinoids, the cell biology of endogenous systems, and the expression of cognate receptors. High-affinity and low-affinity cannabinoid ligands, non-cannabinoid ligands, and receptor subtype-specific antagonists have been developed. In addition, cannabinoid receptor subtype-specific molecular probes and antibodies as well as knockout animals have become available in the last few years. These experimental tools should prove highly useful to basic scientists and clinical researchers as they assess the acute as well as long-term effects of marijuana and cannabinoids on the immune system.

EFFECTS OF CANNABINOIDS ON INFECTIONS

Other than a few early studies on host resistance in mice or guinea pigs to infections with herpes simplex viruses and *Listeria monocytogenes*, there have been few studies of the effects of cannabinoids on infectious diseases. Experimental evidence which links directly the use of cannabis or cannabinoids in a recreational or therapeutic mode to compromised host resistance in humans is not available. Data obtained have been extrapolated from studies performed on experimental animals or using *in vitro* culture systems.

Arata et al. (1992) reported that THC affects macrophage functional activities *in vitro* against *Legionella pneumophila*, the causative agent of Legionnaires' disease. Treatment of macrophages from A/J mice with THC resulted in enhanced growth of *Legionella* within macrophages. In addition, THC treatment overcame macrophage restriction of the growth of *Legionella* that is normally induced by macrophage activation with bacterial lipopolysaccharide. Klein et al. (1994) extended these studies to demonstrate that THC induces significantly increased mortality in mice infected with *Legionella*. *Legionella*-primed mice challenged with a secondary lethal dose survived the challenge infection. However, significantly increased mortality was obtained in animals subjected to the same *Legionella* infection and challenge regimen but receiving THC three weeks prior to the *Legionella* exposure. Kusher et al. (1994) assessed the effect of THC on the synthesis of tumor necrosis factor alpha (TNFα) by human large granular lymphocytes (LGL) in culture. These investigators reported that THC at physiological levels down-regulated TNFα production and diminished LGL cytolytic activity against K562 tumor cells. Based on these studies, it was suggested that, since the NK/polymorphonuclear neutrophil axis represents an important early defense against the opportunistic fungus *Candida albicans,* repression of this system by THC could contribute to susceptibility to infections with opportunistic pathogens.

The few studies performed to assess the effects of marijuana or cannabinoids on resistance to infection in humans have yielded contradictory results. Gross et al. (1991) reported that marijuana consumption altered responsiveness of human papillomavirus (HPV) to systemic recombinant interferon alpha 2a treatment. Simeon et al. (1996) examined characteristics of Jamaicans who smoked marijuana before sex and their risk status for sexually transmitted diseases. The results of a national sample of 2580 randomly selected individuals administered a questionnaire indicated that more persons who smoked marijuana before sex had a history of sexually transmitted diseases than non-marijuana smokers. The difference was significant among men, but not among women. The investigators indicated that, although it was not possible to establish whether the association was causal, there was an increased risk for sexually transmitted diseases among men who smoked marijuana before sex.

On the other hand, Miller and Goodridge (2000) undertook a retrospective study to evaluate the relationship between marijuana use and sexually transmitted diseases in pregnant women. Examination of clinical records over a twelve and one-half month period of 86 women entering prenatal care, and who used no illicit substance other than marijuana, was compared with that of 441 drug-free women. No significant differences in the prevalence of gonorrhea, chlamydia, syphilis, human immunodeficiency virus, hepatitis B virus, human papilloma virus, or herpes virus were noted. Also, no differences were found for prevalence of more than one infectious agent. It was concluded that marijuana use was not associated with sexually transmitted disease in pregnant women.

In contrast to the equivocal results obtained for marijuana and susceptibility to infections, Bass et al. (1996) indicated that a synthetic non-psychotropic cannabinoid could prove useful in the treatment of bacterial infection. The synthetic non-psychotropic cannabinoid dexanabinol (HU-211), when used in combination with antimicrobial therapy, was effective in reducing brain damage in a rat model of pneumococcal meningitis. Brain edema and blood-brain barrier impairment were significantly reduced for infected animals receiving combination ceftriaxone and HU-211 therapy as compared with control animal groups.

EFFECTS OF CANNABINOIDS ON IMMUNE CELLS

Effects of cannabis and cannabinoids on host resistance to infections have occurred in association with changes in cellular and humoral immunity, suggesting a functional linkage between these two events. Studies conducted since the early 1970s reported that cannabinoids and marijuana affect the functions of various immune cells from rodents and humans including B lymphocytes (Zimmerman et al. 1977; Smith et al. 1978; Baczynsky and Zimmerman 1983; Klein and Friedman 1990; Nahas and Osserman 1991; Kaminski et al. 1992), T lymphocytes (Nahas et al. 1974; Gupta et al. 1974; Peterson et al. 1976; Nahas et al. 1977; Klein et al. 1985; Cabral et al. 1987; Klein et al. 1991; Lee et al.1995), macrophages (Mann et al. 1971; Drath et al. 1979; Lopez-Cepero et al. 1986; Cabral and Mishkin 1989; Burstein et al. 1994), and natural killer (NK) cells (Specter et al. 1986; Patel et al. 1985; Klein et al. 1987; Kawakami et al. 1988).

Cannabinoids may affect the immune system by altering functional capabilities of immunocytes rather than affecting their relative numbers or distribution. Del Arco et al. (2000) exposed Wistar rats to the potent synthetic cannabinoid agonist HU-210 during gestation and lactation. It was found that perinatal exposure partially affected the distribution of lymphocyte subpopulations in the spleen and peripheral blood. HU-210 treatment resulted in a reduction of T-helper cells in the spleen and in a dose-related decrease in the ratio of T-helper/T-cytotoxic lymphocytes in peripheral blood. In addition, animals exhibited decreased responsiveness of the hypothalamic-pituitary-adrenal (HPA) axis. Basal levels of luteinizing hormone (LH) were elevated in animals receiving HU-210 while those for corticosterone were reduced. The investigators concluded that maternal exposure to cannabinoids resulted in minor changes in the development of the immune system, but could induce long-lasting alterations in the functional status of the HPA axis.

Baldwin et al. (1997) evaluated the function of human alveolar macrophages recovered from the lungs of nonsmokers and habitual smokers of tobacco, marijuana, or crack cocaine. Macrophages recovered from marijuana smokers were deficient in their ability to phagocytose *Staphylococcus aureus*, and were severely limited in the capacity to kill bacteria and tumor cells. Experiments in which NG-monomethyl-L-arginine monoacetate, an inhibitor of nitric oxide synthase, was used suggested that macrophages from marijuana smokers were not able to use nitric oxide (NO) as an antibacterial effector molecule. Furthermore, macrophages from marijuana smokers, but not from smokers of tobacco or cocaine, produced lower levels of TNFα, granulocyte/macrophage colony-stimulating factor (GMC-SF), and interleukin-6 (IL-6) when stimulated with lipopolysaccharide in culture when compared with alveolar macrophages obtained from control subjects. Based on these observations, it was concluded that habitual exposure of the lung to marijuana impaired select functions of alveolar macrophages including their capacity to produce cytokines.

McCoy et al. (1995) assessed the ability of macrophages and macrophage-like cells exposed to THC to process and present soluble protein. THC was found to exert a differential effect on the capacity of macrophages to process antigens that are necessary for CD4+ T lymphocytes. THC inhibited the processing of hen egg lysozyme (HEL), augmented that of cytochrome *c*, and had no apparent effect on processing of ovalbumin. It was concluded that the nature of the effect of THC on antigen processing was dependent on the intrinsic conformation of the antigen itself. Matveyeva et al. (2000) extended these studies to demonstrate that the THC induced impairment of HEL processing was due, at least in part, to a selective increase in aspartyl cathepsin D proteolytic activity. It was suggested that upregulation of cathepsin D activity resulted in "over-processing" of HEL yielding peptides below the critical size required for antigen presentation. In addition, Clements et al. (1996) demonstrated that THC also suppressed a fixation-resistant co-stimulatory signal to helper T cells by diminishing expression of macrophage heat-stable antigen.

EFFECTS OF CANNABINOIDS ON CYTOKINES

A mode of action by which cannabinoids affect immunocyte functional activities, may be their capacity to express and process effector molecules, including chemokines and cytokines. Newton et al. (1998) demonstrated that the addition of THC to murine splenocytes stimulated with pokeweed mitogen (PWM) resulted in increased levels of the cytokines interleukin-4 (IL-4) and interleukin-10 (IL-10), which are associated with Th2 responses. In contrast, THC treatment resulted in decreased levels of interferon gamma (IFNγ), interleukin-15 (IL-15), and interleukin-12 (IL-12), which are associated with Th1 responses. Thus, cannabinoids induced a shift in the expression of lymphocyte cytokines associated with cell-mediated immunity (i.e., Th1) versus humoral immunity (i.e., Th2). These investigators indicated also that macrophages produced a factor that was responsible for the IL-4 increase, suggesting that macrophages play a role in the Th1 versus Th2 effects. Furthermore, peritoneal macrophages directly exposed to THC and cultured in the presence of various stimulators exhibited decreased production of IL-12, IL-15, and IL-6 while demonstrating increased production of interleukin-1 alpha (IL-1α), interleukin-1 beta (IL-1β), and TNFα. The results suggest that THC affects macrophages in splenocyte cultures and that these cells, as well as lymphocytes, are involved in alterations in levels of cytokines.

Srivastava et al. (1998) used human T, B, eosinophilic, and CD8+ NK cell lines as *in vitro* models to examine the effects of exposure to THC or the relatively non-psychotropic cannabinoid cannabidiol (CBD) on the production of cytokines and of constitutively-expressed, as well as inducibly-expressed chemokines. It was found that cannabinoids exerted a multiplicity of alterations in levels of cytokines from various immune cells. These effects were neither uniform in action nor consistent across cell lineages. THC decreased the constitutive production of the CXC chemokine interleukin-8 (IL-8), of the CC chemokines macrophage inflammatory protein-1 alpha (MIP-1α), inflammatory protein-1 beta (MIP-1β), and Regulated on Activation Normal T Cell Expressed and Secreted (RANTES) protein, and of phorbol ester-stimulated production of TNFα, GM-CSF, and IFNγ by NK cells. THC also inhibited the expression of MIP-1β in human T-lymphotropic virus 1 (HTLV-1)-positive B lymphocytes. In contrast, THC treatment resulted in augmented levels of IL-8, MIP-1α, and MIP-1β in B lymphocytes and IL-8 and MIP-1β in eosinophils. Both CBD and THC inhibited the production of IL-10 in HUT-78 T cells.

Klein et al. (1993) were among the first to relate cannabinoid effects on levels of cytokines to a specific disease process. They reported that THC induces cytokine-mediated mortality of mice infected with *Legionella*. Mice receiving THC, before and after a sublethal injection of *Legionella*, experienced acute collapse and death. The THC-induced mortality resembled cytokine-mediated shock. Acute phase sera from THC-treated animals contained significantly elevated levels of TNF and IL-6 implicating these cytokines as causative, at least in part, of the enhanced mortalities. Mice receiving a normally sub-lethal injection of *Legionella* and administered anti-TNFα, anti-IL-6, or a mixture of anti-IL-1α and anti-IL-1β antibodies before the second THC injection, were protected from THC-induced mortalities. Antibodies against IL-6 were shown to be the most effective in rendering protection. Subsequent experiments performed on cultured splenocytes obtained from mice infected with *Legionella* and administered THC demonstrated alterations in levels of cytokines that were attributable to T lymphocyte subsets (Newton et al. 1994). Splenocytes from THC-treated infected animals stimulated in culture with mitogen were deficient in IFNγ production. In addition, increased production of antibody to *Legionella* of the IgG_1 isotype, as compared to that for the IgG_{2a} isotype, was observed in sera of infected mice treated with THC. Furthermore, THC treatment of cultured, normal splenocytes stimulated with mitogen resulted in production of relatively higher levels of IL-4 as compared with those for IFNγ. In additional studies, Klein et al. (2000) reported that THC treatment of mice suppressed early IFNγ, IL-12, and IL-12 receptor beta 2 responses to *Legionella pneumophila* infection. The Th2-promoting cytokine, IL-4, was increased upon infection with *Legionella* and this increase was augmented following THC administration. However, it was suggested that suppression of Th1 immunity to *Legionella* was not due to an increase in production of IL-4 but rather to a decrease in that of IFNγ and IL-12. Collectively, the studies performed using *Legionella* as an infectivity model suggest that cannabinoids cause a disruption of the network of cytokines which results in a shift from Th1 to Th2 lymphocyte subtype activity. This cannabinoid-mediated shift in Th1 versus Th2 cytokine activity could explain exacerbated infection with *Legionella*.

Massi et al. (1998) also noted that THC could cause alterations in the expression profile of cytokines. These investigators examined the effect of acute versus chronic subcutaneous administration of THC on immune functional and biochemical parameters in male Swiss mice. It was reported that acute exposure to THC had no effect on the splenocyte proliferative response to concanavalin A or on NK cell activity. However, a significant decrease in interleukin-2 (IL-2) production was noted. Chronic administration, for which mice were shown to be tolerant to THC-induced analgesia, resulted in inhibition of the splenocyte proliferative response, diminished NO activity, and reduction in levels of IL-2 and IFNγ.

Recent studies suggest that, in addition to cannabinoids, various endogenous fatty acid ethanolamides participate in the regulation of cytokine responses. Berdyshev et al. (1997) compared the effect of anandamide (arachidonic acid ethanolamide), palmitoylethanolamide, and THC on the production of TNFα, IL-4, IL-6, IL-8, IL-10, and IFNγ by stimulated human peripheral blood mononuclear cells. Anandamide diminished the production of IL-6 and IL-8 at nanomolar concentrations but inhibited that of TNFα, IFNγ, and IL-4 at micromolar concentrations. Palmitoylethanolamide inhibited production of IL-4, IL-6, and IL-8 at concentrations similar to those of anandamide but had no effect on TNFα and IFNγ. THC exerted a biphasic effect on the production of cytokines. Maximal inhibition of TNFα, IL-6, and IL-8 occurred at nanomolar levels. However, at micromolar concentrations, THC caused an augmentation of levels of TNFα, IL-6, and IL-8 as well as IFNγ. Molina-Holgado et al. (1997) demonstrated that the endogenous cannabinoid anandamide suppressed NO and TNFα production by primary cultures of neonatal BALB/c mouse cortical astrocytes in response to exposure to Theiler's virus (TMEV) or bacterial lipopolysaccharide (LPS). These investigators suggested that anandamide might play an immunoregulatory role in the central nervous system (CNS).

Collectively, studies indicate that exogenous as well as endogenous cannabinoids affect the response profile for cytokines and that the nature of alterations is dependent on the concentration of cannabinoid applied. Immunomodulatory effects of cannabinoids on the production of cytokines may vary also as a function of age. Ramarathinam et al. (1997) reported that THC exerted a differential modulation of cytokines by lymphoid cells from young versus old mice. IL-4 and IL-10 production by lymphoid cells of older mice treated with THC was consistently up-regulated in response to stimulation with concanavalin A or anti-CD3 antibody. These observations suggest that aging may be an important variable for consideration when assessing immunomodulatory effects of cannabinoids.

The data indicating that cannabinoids can alter the expression profile of cytokines also suggest a potential for these compounds as selective modulators of pathological inflammatory processes. That is, since cannabinoids have the capacity to diminish the production of cytokines, appropriately designed analogs devoid of psychotropic properties could serve as therapeutic agents applicable of the treatment of disease marked by chronic or exacerbated production of cytokines. In this context, Shohami et al. (1997) reported that HU-211 exhibited pharmacological properties of an N-methyl-D-aspartate (NMDA)-receptor antagonist and acted as an effective cerebroprotectant in an experimental model of traumatic brain injury. The experimental model for closed head injury (CHI) exhibited edema, blood-brain-barrier disruption, motor and memory dysfunction as well as spatial and temporal induction of markers for the cytokines IL-1, IL-6, and TNFα. HU-211 exerted an inhibitory effect on TNFα production by affecting its post-translational maturation. It was suggested that, since cytokines may play a role in the pathophysiology of brain injury, TNF-modulating agents such as HU-211 could serve to improve final neurological outcome if administered within an early time frame following CHI. Gallily et al. (1997) extended these studies to demonstrate that HU-211 also has the ability to rescue rodents from endotoxic shock after LPS injection. HU-211 administered to BALB/c mice prior to introduction of LPS resulted in a significant reduction in lethality. Furthermore, administration of HU-211 to Sprague-Dawley rats prior to treatment with LPS abolished the typical hypotensive response resulting from administration of endotoxin. In addition, HU-211 had a marked inhibitory effect on the ability of murine peritoneal macrophages and rat alveolar macrophages maintained in culture to produce TNFα and NO in response to LPS. These data suggest that HU-211 may have therapeutic potential in the treatment of TNFα-mediated pathologies. Achiron et al. (2000) indicated that HU-211 also reduces the inflammatory response in the brain and spinal cord in rats used as experimental models of autoimmune encephalomyelitis. It was suggested from these studies that HU-211 might be useful as an alternative mode of treatment of acute relapses of multiple sclerosis. In addition to the synthetic compound HU-211, the nonpsychoactive cannabis constituent cannabidiol (CBD) has been reported to act as an oral anti-arthritic therapeutic in a murine model of collagen-induced arthritis (CIA) (Malfait et al. 2000). CBD administered after the onset of clinical symptoms effectively blocked progression of arthritis and was equally effective when administered intraperitoneally or orally. Furthermore, clinical improvement was accompanied by protection of the joints against severe damage. It was postulated that CBD through its combined immunosuppressive and anti-inflammatory actions has a potent anti-arthritic effect on CIA.

MECHANISMS BY WHICH MARIJUANA AND CANNABINOIDS ALTER IMMUNE FUNCTION

Cannabis and cannabinoids exert a wide range of *in vivo* and *in vitro* effects on immune cells. Cannabinoids exert augmenting (McCoy et al. 1995; Derocq et al. 1995; Srivastava et al. 1998) as well as inhibitory effects of immune cell functions (reviewed in: Munson et al. 1976; Cabral and Dove Pettit 1998). Pross et al. (1992) reported that THC exerts concentration-dependent biphasic effects on immune cells. These investigators assessed the effect of THC on T lymphocyte stimulation with anti-CD3 antibody and revealed that lower drug concentrations increased proliferation while higher concentrations inhibited the response. Concentration-dependent augmenting effects of cannabinoids have also been observed by Derocq et al. (1995). It was reported that human tonsillar B-cells exposed to nanomolar concentrations of cannabinoid exhibited enhanced growth and that this enhancement was inhibited by pertussis toxin suggesting that a G protein-coupled receptor process was involved. The observation that SR141716A, an antagonist specific for the CB_1 cannabinoid receptor (Rinaldi-Carmona et al. 1994), had no effect on the cannabinoid-mediated increased proliferative response along with the identification of large amounts of CB_2 receptor mRNA in human B cells, suggested that the growth enhancing activity was mediated through the CB_2 cannabinoid receptor. Biphasic effects of cannabinoids with respect to immune cell lineages have been observed by Klein et al. (1985). These investigators demonstrated that THC concentrations in the micromolar range suppressed mouse splenocyte proliferation to T cell mitogens and to the B cell mitogen LPS. However, B cells appeared to be more sensitive than T cells to the effects of THC.

Cannabinoids may alter immune cell activities by multiple modes of action. At high concentrations (i.e., 10^{-5} M or greater), THC and other cannabinoids can cause membrane perturbation and disruption. Relatively high concentrations which would account for such effects are achievable in humans in the context of immune cells which populate and circulate through the lung, an organ which would be exposed directly to marijuana smoke and hence to relatively high concentrations of exogenous cannabinoids. Physical disruption of cellular membranes could affect protein translational and post-translational events of immune cell effector molecules. Furthermore, since cannabinoids such as THC are highly lipophilic, their interaction with cellular membranes could alter membrane fluidity with consequent alterations in selective permeability (Wing et al. 1985). Such alterations in membranes may account for the reported inhibition of protein synthesis (Cabral and Mishkin 1989; Cabral and Fischer-Stenger 1994) and of molecular precursor transport by THC (Desoize et al. 1979). At lower concentrations, and at sites distal to the lung, cannabinoids may affect immune cell functions by signaling through cannabinoid receptors. Such receptors have been identified both within the brain and on cells of the immune system. The CB_1 was the first cannabinoid receptor to be identified and has been localized to neuronal tissues (Matsuda et al.1990) and testis (Galiègue et al. 1995), and to a lesser extent to immune cells (Galiègue et al. 1995; Waksman et al. 1999). The second cannabinoid receptor, the CB_2 has been observed in cells of the immune system (Munro et al. 1993; Bouaboula et al. 1993; Galiègue et al. 1995; Facci et al. 1995). Both receptors are coupled to a pertussis toxin-sensitive G_i/G_o protein (Howlett and Fleming 1984; Howlett 1985; Howlett et al. 1986; Matsuda et al. 1990). Binding of cannabinoid ligand to cannabinoid receptors results in an increase in the affinity of GTP for the $G\alpha$ subunit of the G protein, a decrease in affinity for GDP, and dissociation of the subunit from the G protein complex. The dissociated $G\alpha$ subunit interacts with adenylate cyclase to inhibit its activity resulting in decreases in levels of the second messenger cAMP (Howlett 1984; Howlett et al. 1990; Felder et al. 1992; Felder et al. 1995) and initiation of mitogen-activated protein kinase (MAPK) and immediate early gene signaling pathways (Bouaboula et al. 1993, 1995, 1996). In turn, the $\beta\gamma$ complex of the G protein can interact with phospholipase C leading to release of inositol-tris-phosphate (IP_3), activation of IP_3-gated calcium channels, and release of Ca^{++} from intracellular stores (Netzeband et al. 1999). The $\beta\gamma$ complex also can activate protein kinase B through class-1_B phosphoinositide 3' kinases (Gomez Del Pulgar et al. 2000). A similar series of events occurs for the CB_2 cannabinoid receptor except that, in contrast to the CB_1, no modulation of N-type calcium channels (Mackie and Hille 1992) has been observed (Felder et al. 1995). Thus, interaction of cannabinoid ligands with cannabinoid receptors can activate different signal transduction pathways that could affect a diverse array of cellular functions.

The presence of CB_2 receptors within immune cells suggests a role for these receptors in their functional activities. Transcripts (i.e., mRNAs) for the CB_2 have been found in spleen and tonsils (Galiègue et al. 1995; Munro et al. 1993) and other immune tissues and cells (Munro et al. 1993; Bouaboula et al. 1993). However, in all studies reported to date, levels of message for the CB_2 have been found to exceed those for the CB_1. The distribution pattern of levels of CB_2 mRNA displays major variation in human blood cell populations with a rank order of B lymphocytes > NK cells > monocytes > polymorphonuclear neutrophils > T8 lymphocytes > T4 lymphocytes (Galiègue et al. 1995). A rank order for levels of CB_2 transcripts similar to that for primary human cell types has been recorded for human cell lines belonging to the myeloid, monocytic, and lymphoid lineages (Galiègue et al. 1995). In addition, the presence of cognate protein has been demonstrated in rat lymph nodes, Peyer's patches, and spleen (Lynn and Herkenham 1994). The differential levels of cannabinoid receptors reported for different immune cell types may account, at least in part, for the distinctive levels of sensitivity to cannabinoid mediated action on the part of immunocytes of different lineages.

Initial studies to examine the role of cannabinoid receptors in cannabinoid-mediated alteration of immune cell activities were primarily of an implicative nature. Kaminski et al. (1992, 1994) noted that suppression of the humoral immune response by cannabinoids was mediated partially by inhibition of adenylate cyclase through a pertussis toxin sensitive guanine nucleotide binding protein (G protein) coupled mechanism, implicating a cannabinoid receptor in this process. THC and the synthetic bicyclic cannabinoid CP55940 inhibited the lymphocyte proliferative response and the sheep erythrocyte IgM antibody-forming cell response of murine splenocytes to phorbol-12-myristate-13-acetate (PMA) plus the calcium ionophore ionomycin. Jeon et al. (1996) suggested that LPS-inducible NO release by the murine macrophage-like cell line RAW264.7 was suppressed by THC and other agonists by mechanisms that involved cannabinoid receptors. Furthermore, attenuation of inducible NO gene expression by THC was reported to be mediated through the inhibition of nuclear factor-κB/Rel activation. In addition, Burstein et al. (1994) presented data indicating that THC-induced arachidonic acid release from mouse peritoneal cells occurred through a series of events consistent with a receptor-mediated process that involved the stimulation of one or more phospholipases.

Recent studies have focused on the definition of the cannabinoid receptor subtype, which may be linked functionally to cannabinoid-mediated alterations in immune cell functions. Waksman et al. (1999) reported that cannabinoids affected the production of inducible NO by neonatal rat microglial cells and that this effect was linked to the CB_1 receptor. The inhibitory effect was stereoselective, consistent with the involvement of a cannabinoid receptor. The dose-dependent inhibition of NO release was exerted by the receptor high affinity binding enantiomer CP55940 while a lower effect for each comparable concentration tested was exerted by the low affinity binding paired enantiomer CP56667. Furthermore, reversal in CP55940-mediated inhibition of NO release was effected when microglial cells were pretreated with the CB_1 receptor-selective antagonist SR141716A consistent with a functional linkage to the CB_1 receptor. Stefano et al. (1996) reported that the CB_1 receptor was linked also to cannabinoid-mediated alterations in the production of constitutive NO. However, in contrast to effects on inducible NO, cannabinoid receptor agonists increased constitutive NO levels in cultures of human monocytes. As in the case of effects on inducible NO, the effect on constitutive NO production was reversed by the CB_1 receptor antagonist SR141716A supporting that the CB_1 receptor was involved in the augmentation process.

Smith et al. (2000) indicated that the CB_1 receptor played a role in the modulation of cytokine production in response to cannabinoid ligands. Two cannabinoid receptor agonists, WIN 55212-2 and HU-210, were examined for their effects on LPS-induced cytokine production in *Corynebacterium parvum* (*C. parvum*)-primed and unprimed mice. Both cannabinoids, when administered to mice before LPS, decreased serum levels of TNFα and IL-12 while increasing those for IL-10. The two agonists also protected *C. parvum*-primed mice against the lethal effects of LPS. These cannabinoid-induced effects on cytokine production were reversed by the CB_1 receptor antagonist SR141716A, but not by the CB_2 receptor-specific antagonist SR144528, consistent with a functional linkage to the CB_1 receptor. Moreover, it was reported that SR141716A when administered alone modulated cytokine responses in a fashion comparable to that of WIN55212-2 and HU-210 suggesting that it could act as a partial agonist of the CB_1 receptor.

There is a larger body of data which supports the CB_2 cannabinoid receptor as linked functionally to cannabinoid-mediated alteration of immune functions. McCoy et al. (1999) implied that a functional linkage existed between cannabinoid-mediated inhibition of antigen processing by macrophages and the CB_2 receptor. In their studies, processing of HEL was inhibited by THC and other cannabinoid agonists. Stereoselective cannabinoid enantiomers showed a differential inhibitory effect for the bioactive enantiomer CP55940 versus that of its less bioactive paired enantiomer CP56667. Furthermore, the CB_1-selective antagonist SR141716A did not block the inhibitory effect of the cannabinoid agonist while the CB_2-selective antagonist SR144528 (Rinaldi-Carmona et al. 1998) did. Zhu et al. (2000) reported that THC inhibits antitumor immunity by a CB_2 receptor-mediated, cytokine-dependent pathway. Accelerated growth of tumor implants was observed following intermittent administration of THC in two weakly immunogenic lung cancer mouse models. In contrast to the results obtained with immunocompetent mice, THC had no effect on tumor growth of implants in severe combined immunodeficiency (SCID) mice. It was demonstrated, in addition, that levels of the immune inhibitory cytokines IL-10 and transforming growth factor beta (TGFβ) were increased at the tumor site as well as in the spleens of mice administered THC. This augmentation was accompanied by a decrease in levels of IFNγ at both sites. The THC-augmentation of tumor growth was prevented by administration of anti-IL-10 or anti-TGFβ neutralizing antibodies. The investigators demonstrated further that administration of the CB_2 cannabinoid receptor antagonist SR144528 blocked the effects of THC. The collective results indicated that THC inhibited antitumor activity and that it did so through a CB_2 cannabinoid receptor-mediated, cytokine-dependent mode.

Derocq et al. (2000) suggested a role for the CB_2 cannabinoid receptor in cell differentiation. These investigators applied Affymetrix DNA chips to the investigation of the gene expression profile of human promyelocytic HL-60 cells transfected with the CB_2 receptor and activated with the synthetic cannabinoid agonist CP55940. Treatment of these cells with CP55940 resulted in activation of a mitogen-activated protein kinase cascade and a receptor desensitization consistent with a functional coupling of the transfected receptors. Activation of the CB_2 receptors at the genomic level effected an up-regulation of genes involved in cytokine synthesis, regulation of transcription, and cell differentiation. A majority of the genes affected were recognized as under the control of nuclear factor-kappa B (NfκB). Many features of the transcriptional events observed by Derocq et al. (2000) appeared to be related to activation of cell differentiation suggesting that the CB_2 receptor plays a role in the initialization of cell maturation. Buckley et al. (2000), employing CB_2 cannabinoid receptor knockout mice to assess the effect of THC on T cell co-stimulation, confirmed the role of the CB_2 cannabinoid receptor as linked functionally to immunomodulation. THC was shown to inhibit helper T cell activation through macrophages derived from wild-type, but not from knockout mice, indicative of at least this immune effect as mediated by the CB_2 receptor. In contrast, central nervous effects of cannabinoids remain unaffected in the knockout mice.

There have been few studies that have addressed the role of cannabinoid receptors in cannabinoid-mediated alterations in resistance to infectious agents. Noe et al. (1998), using syncytial formation as a barometer of infection, reported that cannabinoid receptor agonists enhanced syncytia formation in MT-2 cells infected with cell free human immunodeficiency virus MN strain

implicated the CB_1 receptor as linked func-
Brucella suis growth within macrophages.
141716A effected a dose-dependent inhibi-
ation of this gram-negative bacterium. The
or agonists CP55940 or WIN55212-2 re-
effect. These results suggested that the CB_1
an inhibitor of macrophage infection by the
is.

lls may express both CB_1 and CB_2 receptors,
al transductional pathways may be activated
hus signaling through cannabinoid receptors
l as to immune cell functional events charac-
as inhibition within the same cell. Indeed,
both types of cannabinoid receptors are in-
lytic activity. Inhibition of NK cell activity
y both the CB_1 and the CB_2 antagonists, al-
more effective. These investigators demon-
reversed completely THC-mediated inhibition
tcome was obtained by Klein et al. (2000),
ent suppressed immunity and early IFNγ,
onses to Legionella pneumophila infection.
demonstrated that the suppressive effects
B_2 antagonists, suggesting that suppression
as linked to both cannabinoid receptors. Mc-
istinctive receptor-mediated functional out-
same immune cell type. These investigators
ntrations of THC induced enhancement of
rome c while simultaneously inhibiting that
thermore, cannabinoids may exert their ef-
ceptor-mediated modes within the same cell
trated that cannabinoid agonists stimulated
ted signal transduction pathways. Fibroblast
ted with a recombinant cannabinoid receptor
ressed cannabinoid receptors were used in
the synthetic cannabinoid receptor agonist
ed receptors coupled to the inhibition of
d for the involvement of a cannabinoid re-
P55940 also stimulated the increase of free
lective fashion indicative of the absence of a
id receptor for this cellular activity.

with target immunocytes by a receptor- or
fundamental result is that basic functional

activities of cells are altered which often are mediated through second messenger systems. Herring and Kaminski (1999) indicated that cannabinol (CBN) mediated inhibition of NFκB, cAMP response element (CRE)-binding protein, and IL-2 secretion by phorbol ester plus calcium ionophore (PMA/Io) stimulated thymocytes. CBN decreased CRE and NFκB binding activity that had been induced by PMA/Io. Both a major CRE DNA binding complex comprised of a cAMP response element-binding protein (CREB)-1 homodimer, as well as a minor CREB-1/activating transcription factor (ATF)-2 complex, were inhibited. In addition, CBN diminished the binding activity of PMA/Io-inducible and non-inducible κB DNA binding complexes. In PMA/Io-stimulated thymocytes, CBN effected a decrease in phosphorylation of CREB/ATF nuclear proteins, and prevented phosphorylation-dependent degradation of the NFκB inhibitory protein IκBα. Herring and Kaminski (1999) suggested that these results indicated a functional link between CBN-mediated inhibition of thymocyte functional activities, including IL-2 production, and inhibition of the transcriptional factor activities of complexes in the CREB/ATF and NFκB/Rel families. These studies were extended by Yea et al. (2000) to demonstrate that inhibition of IL-2 production by CBN was mediated through the inhibition of IL-2 gene transcription. Electrophoretic mobility shift assays demonstrated that CBN inhibited the DNA binding activity of nuclear factor of activated-T cells (NF-AT) and activator protein-1 (AP-1) in a time- and concentration-dependent manner in activated EL4 T-cells. Furthermore, the AP-1 activity was reported to be negatively regulated through inhibition of its protein components, *c-fos* and *c-jun* (Faubert and Kaminski 2000). Thus, the CBN inhibited binding to AP-1 containing sites from the IL-2 promoter was due, in part, to decreased nuclear expression of *c-fos* and *c-jun*. In addition, it was reported that the effects of CBN were due to post-translational modification of these phosphoproteins and that CBN inhibited the activation of ERK MAP kinases. Based on these studies, it was concluded that CBN-induced immunosuppression involved a disruption of the ERK signaling cascade. However, whether a cannabinoid receptor is involved in this transductional cascade of events remains unresolved.

CANNABINOIDS, CANNABIS, AND AIDS

Many studies using *in vitro* and *in vivo* models have addressed the effects of cannabinoids and cannabis on host resistance and immunity. However, there have been few studies that have assessed directly the effects of marijuana usage or of cannabinoid administration in humans. The scarcity of data applies particularly to the evaluation of effects of marijuana, used either in a recreational or therapeutic mode, among humans who have immune deficiencies.

Epidemiological studies similar to those that have been performed to assess effects of tobacco have not been carried out in human populations in relation to infection with the human immunodeficiency virus (HIV). The studies performed to date have yielded limited and often contradictory results as to effects of cannabinoids on human immunity and resistance to infection.

Wallace et al. (1998) examined risk factors and outcomes associated with identification of *Aspergillus* in respiratory specimens from individuals with HIV disease as part of a study to evaluate pulmonary complications of HIV infection. It was indicated that a substantially greater proportion of patients with *Aspergillus* as compared with control subjects died during the study. However, the use of cigarettes and marijuana was found not to be associated with *Aspergillus* respiratory infection. In contrast, Johnson et al. (1999) suggested that marijuana smoking could increase the risk of development of sino-orbital aspergillosis in patients with acquired immune deficiency syndrome (AIDS). DiFranco et al. (1996), through the San Francisco Men's Health Study (SFMHS), evaluated the association of specific recreational drugs and alcohol with laboratory predictors of AIDS. Participants in the study were evaluated at entry into the program in 1984 and in the context of the development of AIDS during six years of follow-up. No substantial association could be obtained between the use of marijuana and the development of AIDS among HIV-infected men. Similarly, Timpone et al. (1997) reported that cannabinoid use in a therapeutic mode exerted few deleterious effects, at least as they related to immune competence and resistance to infection. Persaud et al. (1999) conducted a cross-sectional survey among 124 street- and brothel-based female commercial sex workers in Guyana. No statistically significant association was found between HIV infection and marijuana use.

On the other hand, other studies have suggested that cannabinoids or marijuana exert deleterious effects as they relate to HIV infection. Stefano et al. (1998) reported that long-term exposure of human saphenous vein or thoracic artery endothelium to the human immunodeficiency virus (HIV) envelope protein gp120 in concert with morphine and/or anandamide increased endothelial adhesion of monocytes. It was suggested that enhancement of monocyte adherence was a result of desensitization of the endothelium to further NO release after initial exposure to either anandamide or morphine. The investigators suggested that abuse of opiates and/or cannabinoids could result in higher viral load in the central nervous system. Furthermore, they suggested that the increase in monocyte adherence and mobility indicative of a higher level of transmembrane migration could contribute to a more rapid progression of the AIDS. Tindall et al. (1988) conducted immunoepidemiological studies using univariant and multivariant analyses and implied an association between marijuana use and progression of HIV infection. Caiaffa et al. (1994) indicated that smoking illicit drugs such as marijuana, cocaine, or crack, *Pneumocystis ca-*

rinii pneumonia, and immunosuppression increased risk of bacterial pneumonia in HIV-seropositive users. More recently, Whitfield et al. (1997) examined the impact of ethanol and Marinol®/marijuana usage on HIV+/AIDS patients undergoing azidothymidine, azidothymidine/dideoxycytidine, or dideoxyinosine therapy. In HIV+/AIDS patients with the lowest CD4+ counts (those not on DDI monotherapy), utilization of Marinol®/marijuana did not seem to have a deleterious effect. However, Marinol®/marijuana usage was associated with depressed CD4+ counts and elevated amylase levels within the DDI subgroup. Furthermore, Marinol®/marijuana use was associated with declining health status in both the AZT and AZT/DDC groups.

CONCLUSION

The cumulative data obtained through cell culture studies using various immune cell populations extracted from animals or humans, together with those obtained using animal models of infection, are consistent with the proposition that marijuana and cannabinoids alter immune cell function and can exert deleterious effects on resistance to infection in humans. Both receptor- and non-receptor mediated modes of action have been proposed to account for the effects of cannabinoids. However, few controlled longitudinal epidemiological and immunological studies have been undertaken to correlate the immunosuppressive effects of marijuana smoke or cannabinoids on the incidence of infections or viral disease in humans. Clearly, additional investigation to resolve the long-term immunological consequences of cannabinoid and marijuana use as they relate to resistance to infections in humans is warranted. There is also emerging evidence that select cannabinoid compounds, particularly those devoid of psychotropic properties, may be useful for therapeutic application for pathologies characterized by chronic activation of immune cells or imbalance in expression of Th1 versus Th2 cytokines.

REFERENCES

Achiron, A., S. Miron, V. Lavie, R. Margalit, and A. Biegon. 2000. Dexanabinol (HU-211) effect on experimental autoimmune encephalomyelitis: implications for the treatment of acute relapses of multiple sclerosis. *J Neuroimmunol* 102(1):26-31.

Arata, S., C. Newton, T. Klein, and H. Friedman. 1991. Enhanced growth of *Legionella pneumophila* in tetrahydrocannabinol-treated macrophages. *Proc Soc Exp Biol Med* 199:65-7.

Baczynsky, W. O. T., and A. M. Zimmerman. 1983. Effects of delta-9-tetrahydrocannabinol, cannabinol and cannabidiol on the immune system in mice. *In vitro* investigation using cultured mouse splenocytes. *Pharmacology* 26(1):12-9.

Baldwin, G. C., D. P. Tashkin, D. M. Buckley, A. M., Park, S. M., Dubinett, and M. D. Roth. 1997. Marijuana and cocaine impair alveolar macrophage function and cytokine production. *Am J Respir Crit Care Med* 156(5):1606-13.

Bass, R., D. Engelhard, V. Trembovler, and E. Shohami. 1996. A novel nonpsychotropic cannabinoid, HU-211, in the treatment of experimental pneumococcal meningitis. *J Infect Dis* 173:735-8.

Berdyshev, E. V., E. Boichot, N. Germain, N. Allain, J. P. Anger, and V. Lagente. 1997. Influence of fatty acid ethanolamides and delta9-tetrahydrocannabinol on cytokine and arachidonate release by mononuclear cells. *Eur J Pharmacol* 330(2-3): 231-40.

Bouaboula, M., C. Poinot-Chazel, J. Marchand, X. Canat, B. Bourrie, M. Rinaldi-Carmona, B. Calandra, G. Le Fur, and P. Casellas. 1996. Signaling pathway associated with stimulation of CB2 peripheral cannabinoid receptor. Involvement of both mitogen-activated protein kinase and induction of Krox-24 expression. *Eur J Biochem* 237(3):704-11.

Bouaboula, M., C. Poinot-Chazel, B. Bourrie, X. Canat, B. Calandra, M. Rinaldi-Carmona, G. Le Fur, and P. Casellas. 1995. Activation of mitogen-activated protein kinases by stimulation of the central cannabinoid receptor CB1. *Biochem J* 312: 637-41.

Bouaboula, M., M. Rinaldi, P. Carayon, C. Carillon, B. Delpech, D. Shire, G. Le Fur, and P. Casellas. 1993. Cannabinoid receptor expression in human leukocytes. *Eur J Biochem* 214:173-80.

Buckley, N. E., K. L. McCoy, E. Mezey, T. Bonner, A. Zimmer, C. C. Felder, M. Glass, and A. Zimmer. 2000. Immunomodulation by cannabinoids is absent in mice deficient for the cannabinoid CB(2) receptor. *Eur J Pharmacol* 396(2-3):141-9.

Burnette-Curley, D., F. M. Marciano, K. Fischer, and G. A. Cabral. 1993. Delta-9-tetrahydrocannabinol inhibits cell contact-dependent cytotoxicity of *Bacillus* Calmétte-Guérin-activated macrophages. *Int J Immunopharmacol* 15:371-82.

Burstein, S., J. Budrow, M. Debatis, S. A. Hunter, and A. Subramanian. 1994. Phospholipase participation in cannabinoid-induced release of free arachidonic acid. *Biochem Pharmacol* 48:1253-64.

Cabral, G. A., and D. Dove Pettit. 1998. Drugs and immunity: Cannabinoids and their role in decreased resistance to infectious disease. *J Neuroimmunol* 83:116-23.

Cabral, G. A., and K. Fischer-Stenger. 1994. Inhibition of macrophage inducible protein expression by delta-9-tetrahydrocannabinol. *Life Sci* 54:1831-44.

Cabral, G. A., and E. M. Mishkin. 1989. Delta-9-tetrahydrocannabinol inhibits macrophage protein expression in response to bacterial immunomodulators. *J Toxicol Environ Health* 26:175-82.

Cabral, G. A., P. J. McNerney, and E. M. Mishkin. 1987. Effect of micromolar concentrations of delta-9-tetrahydrocannabinol on herpes simplex virus type 2 replication in vitro. *J Toxicol Environ Health* 21(3):277-93.

Cabral, G. A., J. C. Lockmuller, and E. M. Mishkin. 1986a. Delta-9-tetrahydrocannabinol decreases alpha/beta interferon response to herpes simplex virus type 2 in the B6C3F1 mouse. *Proc Soc Exp Biol Med* 181:305-11.

Cabral, G., E. M. Mishkin, F. M. Marciano, R. E. Coleman, L. S. Harris, and A. E. Munson. 1986b. Effect of delta-9-tetrahydrocannabinol on herpes simplex virus type 2 vaginal infection in the guinea pig. *Proc Soc Exp Biol Med* 182:181-6.

Caiaffa, W. T., D. Vlahov, N. M. D. Graham, J. Astemborski, L. Solomon, K. E. Nelson, and A. Munoz. 1994. Drug smoking, *Pneumocystis carinii* pneumonia, and immunosuppression increase risk of bacterial pneumonia in human immunodeficiency virus-seropositive injection drug users. *Am J Respir Crit Care Med* 150: 1493-8.

Childers, S. R., and S. A. Deadwyler. 1996. Role of cyclic AMP in the actions of cannabinoid receptors. *Biochem Pharmacol* 52:819-27.

Clements, D., G. A. Cabral, and K. L. McCoy. 1996. Delta-9-tetrahydrocannabinol selectively inhibits macrophage co-stimulatory activity and down-regulates heat-stable antigen expression. *J Pharmacol Exp Ther* 277:1315-21.

del Arco, I., R. Munoz, F. Rodriguez De Fonseca, L. Escudero, J. L. Martin-Calderon, M. Navarro, and M. A. Villanua. 2000. Maternal exposure to the synthetic cannabinoid HU-210: effects on the endocrine and immune systems of the adult male offspring. *Neuroimmunomodulation* 7(1):16-26.

Derocq, J. M., O. Jbilo, M. Bouaboula, M. Segui, C. Clere, and P. Casellas. 2000. Genomic and functional changes induced by the activation of the peripheral cannabinoid receptor CB2 in the promyelocytic cells HL-60. Possible involvement of the CB2 receptor in cell differentiation. *J Biol Chem* 275(21):15621-8.

Derocq, J. M., M. Segui, J. Marchand, G. Le Fur, and P. Casellas. 1995. Cannabinoids enhance human B-cell growth at low nanomolar concentrations. *FEBS Letters* 369:177-82.

Desoize, B., C. Leger, and G. G. Nahas. 1979. Plasma membrane inhibition of macromolecular precursor transport by THC. *Biochem Pharmacol* 28:1113-8.

Dewey, W. L. 1986. Cannabinoid pharmacology. *Pharmacol Rev* 38(2):151-78.

DiFranco, M. J, H. W. Sheppard, D. J. Hunter, T. D. Tosteson, and M. S. Ascher. 1996. The lack of association of marijuana and other recreational drugs with progression to AIDS in the San Francisco Men's Health Study. *Ann Epidemiol* 6(4):283-9.

Dove Pettit, D. A., D. L. Anders, M. P. Harrison, and G. A. Cabral. 1996. Cannabinoid receptor expression in immune cells. *Adv Exp Med Biol* 402:119-29.

Drath, D. B., J. M. Shorey, L. Price, and G. L. Huber. 1979. Metabolic and functional characteristics of alveolar macrophages recovered from rats exposed to marijuana smoke. *Infect Immun* 25:268-72.

Facci, L., R. Dal Tosso, S. Romanello, A. Buriani, S. D. Skaper, and A. Leon. 1995. Mast cells express a peripheral receptor and differential sensitivity to anandamide and palmitoylethanolamide. *Proc Natl Acad Sci USA* 92:3376-80.

Faubert, B. L., and N. E. Kaminski. 2000. AP-1 activity is negatively regulated by cannabinol through inhibition of its protein components, c-fos and c-jun. *J Leukoc Biol* 67(2):259-66.

Felder, C. C., K. E. Joyce, E. M. Briley, J. Mansouri, K. Mackie, O. Blond, Y. Lai, A. L. Ma, and R. L. Mitchell. 1995. Comparison of the pharmacology and signal transduction of the human cannabinoid CB_1 and CB_2 receptors. *Mol Pharmacol* 48:443-50.

Felder, C. C., J. S. Veluz, H. L. Williams, E. M. Briley, and L. A. Matsuda. 1992. Cannabinoid agonists stimulate both receptor- and non-receptor-mediated signal transduction pathways in cells transfected with and expressing cannabinoid receptor clones. *Mol Pharmacol* 42:838-45.

Fischer-Stenger, K., A. W. Updegrove, and G. A. Cabral. 1992. Delta-9-tetrahydrocannabinol decreases cytotoxic T lymphocyte activity to herpes simplex virus type 1-infected cells. *Proc Soc Exp Biol Med* 200:422-30.

Friedman, H., and T. W. Klein. 1999. Marijuana and immunity. *Sci Med* 6(2):12-21.

Galiègue, S., S. Mary, J. Marchand, D. Dussosoy, D. Carrière, P. Carayon, M. Bouaboula, D. Shire, G. Le Fur, and P. Casellas. 1995. Expression of central and peripheral cannabinoid receptors in human immune tissues and leukocyte subpopulations. *Eur J Biochem* 232:54-61.

Gallily, R., A. Yamin, Y. Waksmann, H. Ovadia, J. Weidenfeld, A. Bar-Joseph, A. Biegon, R. Mechoulam, and E. Shohami. 1997. Protection against septic shock and suppression of tumor necrosis factor alpha and nitric oxide production by dexanabinol (HU-211), a nonpsychotropic cannabinoid. *J Pharmacol Exp Ther* 283(2): 918-24.

Gomez Del Pulgar, T., G. Velasco, and M. Guzman. 2000. The CB1 cannabinoid receptor is coupled to the activation of protein kinase B/Akt. *Biochem J* 347:369-73.

Gross, A., A. Terraza, J. Marchant, M. Bouaboula, S. Ouahrani-Bettache, J. P. Liautard, P. Casellas, and J. Dornand. 2000. A beneficial aspect of a CB1 cannabinoid receptor antagonist: SR141716A is a potent inhibitor of macrophage infection by the intracellular pathogen *Brucella suis*. *J Leukoc Biol* 67(3): 335-44.

Gross, G., A. Roussaki, H. Ikenberg, and N. Dress. 1991. Genital warts do not respond to systemic recombinant interferon alpha-2a treatment during cannabis consumption. *Dermatologica* 183:203-7.

Gupta, G., M. Grieco, and P. Cushman. 1974. Impairment of rosette-forming T-lymphocytes in chronic marihuana smokers. *New Eng J Med* 291:874-6.

Herring, A. C., and N. E. Kaminski. 1999. Cannabinol-mediated inhibition of nuclear factor-kappa B, cAMP response element-binding protein, and interleukin-2 secretion by activated thymocytes. *J Pharmacol Exp Ther* 291(3):1156-63.

Howlett, A. C. 1985. Cannabinoid inhibition of adenylate cyclase. Biochemistry of the response in neuroblastoma cell membranes. *Mol Pharmacol* 27:429-36.

Howlett, A. C. 1984. Inhibition of neuroblastoma adenylate cyclase by cannabinoid and nantradol compounds. *Life Sci* 35:1803-10.

Howlett, A. C., and R. M. Fleming. 1984. Cannabinoid inhibition of adenylate cyclase. Pharmacology of the response in neuroblastoma cell membranes. *Mol Pharmacol* 26:532-8.

Howlett, A. C., T. M. Champion, G. H. Wilken, and R. Mechoulam. 1990. Stereochemical effects of 11-OH-delta 8-tetrahydrocannabinol-dimethylheptyl to inhibit adenyl cyclase and bind to the cannabinoid receptor. *Neuropharmacol* 29:161-5.

Howlett, A. C., J. M. Qualy, and L. L. Khachchatrian. 1986. Involvement of Gi in the inhibition of adenylate cyclase by cannabimimetic drugs. *Mol Pharmacol* 29: 307-13.

Jeon, Y. J., K. H. Yang, J. T. Pulaski, and N. E. Kaminski. 1996. Attenuation of inducible nitric oxide gene expression by Δ9-tetrahydrocannabinol is mediated through the inhibition of nuclear factor-κB/rel activation. *Mol Pharmacol* 50:334-41.

Johnson, T. E., R. R. Casiano, J. W. Kronish, D. T. Tse, M. Meldrum, and W. Chang. 1999. Sino-orbital aspergillosis in acquired immunodeficiency syndrome. *Arch Ophthalmol* 117(1):57-64.

Kaminski, N. E., M. E. Abood, F. K. Kessler, B. R. Martin, and A. R. Schatz. 1992. Identification of a functionally relevant cannabinoid receptor on mouse spleen cells that is involved in cannabinoid-mediated immune modulation. *Mol Pharmacol* 42:736-42.

Kaminski, N. E., W. S. Koh, K. H. Yang, M. Lee, and F. K. Kessler. 1994. Suppression of the humoral immune response by cannabinoids is partially mediated through inhibition of adenylate cyclase by a pertussis toxin-sensitive G-protein coupled mechanism. *Biochem Pharmacol* 48:1899-908.

Kawakami, Y., T. W. Klein, C. Newton, J. Y. Djeu, S. Specter, and H. Friedman. 1988. Suppression of delta-9-tetrahydrocannabinol of interleukin 2-induced lymphocyte proliferation and lymphokine-activated killer cell activity. *Int J Immunopharmacol* 10:485-8.

Klein, T. W., C. A. Newton, N. Nakachi, and H. Friedman. 2000. Delta 9-tetrahydrocannabinol treatment suppresses immunity and early IFN-gamma, IL-12, and IL-12 receptor beta 2 responses to *Legionella pneumophila* infection. *J Immunol* 164(12):6461-6.

Klein, T. W., C. Newton, and H. Friedman. 1994. Resistance to *Legionella pneumophila* suppressed by the marijuana component, tetrahydrocannabinol. *J Infect Dis* 169:1177-9.

Klein, T., C. Newton, R. Widen, and H. Friedman. 1993. Delta-9-tetrahydrocannabinol injection induces cytokine-mediated mortality of mice infected with *Legionella pneumophila*. *J Pharmacol Exp Ther* 267:635-40.

Klein, T. W., Y. Kawakami, C. Newton, and H. Friedman. 1991. Marijuana components supress induction and cytolytic function of murine cytotoxic T cells *in vitro* and *in vivo*. *J Toxicol Environ Health* 32:465-77.

Klein, T. W. and H. Friedman. 1990. *Drugs of abuse and immune function.* In R. R. Watson (Ed.). Boca Raton:CRC Press.

Klein, T. W., C. Newton, and H. Friedman. 1987. Inhibition of natural killer cell function by marijuana components. *J Toxicol Environmental Health* 20:321-32.

Klein, T. W., C. Newton, R. Widen, and H. Friedman. 1985. The effect of delta-9-tetrahydrocannabinol and 11-hydroxy-delta 9-tetrahydrocannabinol on T-lymphocyte and B-lymphocyte mitogen responses. *J Immunopharmacol* 7:451-66.

Klykken, P. C., S. H. Smith, J. A. Levy, R. Razdan, and A. E. Munson. 1977. Immunosuppressive effects of 8,9-epoxyhexahydrocannabinol (EHHC). *J Pharmacol Exp Ther* 201:573-9.

Kusher, D. I., L. O. Dawson, A. C. Taylor, and J. Y. Djeu. 1994. Effect of the psychoactive metabolite of marijuana, delta-9-tetrahydrocannabinol (THC), on the synthesis of tumor necrosis factor by large granular lymphocytes. *Cellular Immunol* 154(1):99-108.

Lee, M., K. H.Yang, and N. E. Kaminski. 1995. Effects of putative receptor ligands, anandamide and 2-arachidonyl-glycerol, on immune function in B6C3F1 mouse splenocytes. *J Pharmacol Exp Ther* 275:529-36.

Lopez-Cepero, M., M. Friedman, T. Klein, and H. Friedman. 1986. Tetrahydro-cannabinol-induced suppression of macrophage spreading and phagocyte activity *in vitro. J Leukoc Biol* 39: 679-86.

Lynn, A. B., and M. Herkenham. 1994. Localization of cannabinoid receptors and nonsaturable high-density cannabinoid binding sites in peripheral tissues of the rat: implications for receptor-mediated immune modulation by cannabinoids. *J Pharmacol Exp Ther* 268:1612-23.

Mackie, K., and B. Hille. 1992. Cannabinoids inhibit N-type calcium channels in neuroblastoma-glioma cells. *Proc Natl Acad Sci USA* 89:3825-9.

Malfait, A. M., R. Gallily, P. F. Sumariwalla, A. S. Malik, E. Andreakos, R. Mechoulam, and M. Feldmann. 2000. The nonpsychoactive cannabis constituent cannabidiol is an oral anti-arthritic therapeutic in murine collagen-induced arthritis. *Proc Natl Acad Sci USA* 97(17):9561-6.

Mann, P. E. G., A. B. Cohen, T. N. Finley, and A. J. Ladman. 1971. Alveolar macrophages. Structural and functional differences between non-smokers and smokers of marijuana *in vitro. Lab Invest* 25:111-20.

Massi, P., D. Fuzio, D. Vigano, P. Sacerdote, and D. Parolaro. 2000. Relative involvement of cannabinoid CB(1) and CB(2) receptors in Delta(9)-tetrahydrocanna-binol-induced inhibition of natural killer activity. *Eur J Pharmacol* 387(3):343-7.

Massi, P., P. Sacerdote, W. Ponti, D. Fuzio, B. Manfredi, D. Vigano, T. Rubino, M. Bardotti, and D. Parolaro. 1998. Immune function alterations in mice tolerant to delta-9-tetrahydrocannabinol: functional and biochemical parameters. *J Neuroimmunol* 92(1-2):60-6.

Matsuda, L. A., S. J. Lolait, M. J. Brownstein, A. C. Young, and T. I. Bonner. 1990. Structure of a cannabinoid receptor and functional expression of the cloned cDNA. *Nature* 346:561-4.

Matveyeva, M., C. B. Hartman, M. T. Harrison, G. A. Cabral, and K. L. McCoy. 2000. Delta (9)-tetrahydrocannabinol selectively increases aspartyl cathepsin D proteolytic activity and impairs lysozyme processing by macrophages. *Int J Immunopharmacol* 22(5):373-81.

McCoy, K. L., D. Gainey, and G. A. Cabral. 1995. Δ^9-Tetrahydrocannabinol modulates antigen processing by macrophages. *J Pharmacol Exp Ther* 273:1216-23.

McCoy, K. L., M. Matveyeva, S. J. Carlisle, and G. A. Cabral. 1999. Cannabinoid inhibition of the processing of intact lysozyme by macrophages: Evidence for CB2 receptor participation. *J Pharmacol Exp Ther* 289:1620-5.

Miller, J. M. Jr., and C. Goodridge. 2000. Antenatal marijuana use is unrelated to sexually transmitted infections during pregnancy. *Infect Dis Obstet Gynecol* 8(3-4):155-7.

Mishkin, E. M., and G. Cabral. 1985. Delta-9-tetrahydrocannabinol decreases host resistance to herpes simplex virus type 2 vaginal infection in the $B_6C_3F_1$ mouse. *J Gen Virol* 66:2539-49.

Molina-Holgado, F., A. Lledo, and C. Guaza. 1997. Anandamide suppresses nitric oxide and TNF-alpha responses to Theiler's virus or endotoxin in astrocytes. *Neuroreport* 8(8):1929-33.

Morahan, P. S., P. C. Klykken, S. H. Smith, L. S. Harris, and A. E. Munson 1979. Effects of cannabinoids on host resistance to *Listeria monocytogenes* and herpes simplex virus. *Inf Immun* 23:670-4.

Munro, S., K. L. Thomas, and M. Abu-Shaar. 1993. Molecular characterization of a peripheral receptor for cannabinoids. *Nature* 365:61-5.

Munson, A. E., J. A. Levy, L. S. Harris, and W. L. Dewey. 1976. Effects of delta 9-tetrahydrocannabinol on the immune system. *The Pharmacology of Marijuana.* Braude, M. C., and S. Szara. New York: Raven Press.

Munson, A. E., and K. O. Fehr.1983. Immunological Effects of Cannabis. *Cannabis and Health Hazards.* Fehr, K. O. and H. Kalant. Toronto: Alcoholism and Drug Addiction Research Foundation.

Nahas, G. G., A. Morishima, and B. Desoize. 1977. Effects of cannabinoids on macromolecular synthesis and replication of cultured lymphocytes. *Fed Proc* 36:1748-52.

Nahas, G. G., and E. F. Osserman. 1991. Altered serum immunoglobulin concentration in chronic marijuana smokers. *Adv Exp Med Biol* 288:25-32.

Nahas, G. G., N. Suciu-Foca, J. P. Armand, and A. Morishima 1974. Inhibition of cellular mediated immunity in marihuana smokers. *Science* 183:419-20.

Netzeband, J. G., S. M. Conroy, K. L. Parsons, and D. L. Gruol. 1999. Cannabinoids enhance NMDA-elicited Ca^{2+} signals in cerebellar granule neurons in culture. *J Neurosci* 19:8765-77.

Newton, C., T. Klein, and H. Friedman. 1998. The role of macrophages in THC-induced alteration of the cytokine network. *Adv Exp Med Biol* 437:207-14.

Newton, C. A., T. W. Klein, and H. Friedman. 1994. Secondary immunity to *Legionella pneumophila* and Th1 activity are suppressed by delta-9-tetrahydrocannabinol injection. *Inf Immun* 62:4015-20.

Noe, S. N., S. B. Nyland, K. Ugen, H. Friedman, and T. W. Klein. 1998. Cannabinoid receptor agonists enhance syncytia formation in MT-2 cells infected with cell free HIV-1MN. *Adv Exp Med Biol* 437:223-9.

Patel, V., M. Borysenko, M. S. A. Kumar, and W. J. Millard. 1985. Effects of acute and subchronic delta-9-tetrahydrocannabinol administration on the plasma catecholamine, beta-endorphin, and corticosterone levels and splenic natural killer cell activity in rats. *Proc Soc Exp Biol Med* 180:400-4.

Persaud, N. E., W. Klaskala, T. Tewari, J. Schultz, and M. Baum. 1999. Drug use and syphilis. Co-factors for HIV transmission among commercial sex workers in Guyana. *West Indian Med J* 48(2):52-6.

Peterson, B. H., J. Graham, and L. Lemberger. 1976. Marihuana, tetrahydrocannabinol and T-cell function. *Life Sci* 19:395-400.

Pross, S. H., Y. Nakano, R. Widen, S. McHugh, C. A. Newton, T. W. Klein, and H. Friedman. 1992. Differing effects of delta-9-tetrahydrocannabinol (THC) on murine spleen cell populations dependent upon stimulators. *Int J Immunopharmacol* 14:1019-27.

Ramarathinam, L., S. Pross, O. Plescia, C. Newton, R. Widen, and H. Friedman. 1997. Differential immunologic modulatory effects of tetrahydrocannabinol as a function of age. *Mech Ageing Dev* 96(1-3):117-26.

Rinaldi-Carmona, M., F. Barth, M. Héaulme, D. Shire, B. Calandra, C. Congy, S. Martinez, J. Maruani, G. Néliat, D. Caput, P. Ferrara, P. Soubrié, J. C. Breliére, and G. Le Fur. 1994. Sr141716A, a potent and selective antagonist of the brain cannabinoid receptor. *FEBS Letters* 350:240-4.

Rinaldi-Carmona, M., F. Barth, J. Millan, J. M. Derocq, P. Casellas, C. Congy, D. Oustric, M. Sarran, M. Bouaboula, B. Calandra, M. Portier, D. Shire, J. C. Breliére, and G. Le Fur. 1998. SR144528, the first potent and selective antagonist of the CB2 cannabinoid receptor. *J Pharmacol Exp Ther* 284:644-50.

Shohami, E., R. Gallily, R. Mechoulam, R. Bass, and T. Ben-Hur. 1997. Cytokine production in the brain following closed head injury: dexanabinol (HU-211) is a novel TNF-alpha inhibitor and an effective neuroprotectant. *J Neuroimmunol* 72(2): 169-77.

Simeon, D. T., B. Bain, G. E. Wyatt, E. LeFranc, H. Ricketts, C. C. Chambers, and M. B. Tucker. 1996. Characteristics of Jamaicans who smoke marijuana before sex and their risk status for sexually transmitted diseases. *West Indian Med J* 45(1):9-13.

Smith, S. R., C. Terminelli, and G. Denhardt. 2000. Effects of cannabinoid receptor agonist and antagonist ligands on production of inflammatory cytokines and anti-inflammatory interleukin-10 in endotoxemic mice. *J Pharmacol Exp Ther* 293(1): 136-50.

Smith, S. H., L. S. Harris, I. M. Uwaydah, and A. E. Munson. 1978. Structure-activity relationships of natural and synthetic cannabinoids in suppression of humoral and cell-mediated immunity. *J Pharmacol Exp Ther* 207:165-70.

Specter, S. C., T. W. Klein, C. Newton, M. Mondragon, R. Widen, and H. Friedman. 1986. Marijuana effects on immunity:suppression of human natural killer cell activity by delta-9-tetrahydrocannabinol. *Int J Immunopharmacol* 8:741-5.

Specter, S., G. Lancz, G. Westrich, and H. Friedman. 1991. Delta-9-tetrahydrocannabinol augments murine retroviral induced immunosuppression and infection. *Int J Immunopharmacol* 13:411-7.

Srivastava, M. D., B. I. Srivastava, and B. Brouhard. 1998. Delta-9-tetrahydrocannabinol and cannabidiol alter cytokine production by human immune cells. *Immunopharmacology* 40(3):179-85.

Stefano, G. B., M. Salzet, and T. V. Bilfinger. 1998. Long-term exposure of human blood vessels to HIV gp120, morphine, and anandamide increases endothelial adhesion of monocytes: uncoupling of nitric oxide release. *J Cardiovasc Pharmacol* 31(6):862-8.

Stefano, G. B., Y. Liu, and M. S. Goligorsky. 1996. Cannabinoid receptors are coupled to nitric oxide release in invertebrate immunocytes, microglia, and human monocytes. *J Biol Chem* 271: 19238-42.

Timpone, J. G., D. J. Wright, N. Li, M. J. Egorin, M. E. Enama, J. Mayers, and J. Galetto. 1997. The safety and pharmokinetics of single-agent and combination therapy with Megestrol acetate and Dronabinol for the treatment of HIV wasting syndrome. *AIDS Res Hum Retroviruses* 13:305-15.

Tindall, B., D. A. Cooper, B. Donovan, T. Barnes, C. R. Philpot, J. Gold, and R. Penny. 1988. The Sydney AIDS Project: development of acquired immunodeficiency syndrome in a group of HIV seropositive homosexual men. *Aust N Z J Med* 18(1):8-15.

Waksman, Y., J. M. Olson, S. J. Carlisle, and G. A. Cabral. 1999. The central cannabinoid receptor (CB1) mediates inhibition of nitric oxide production by rat microglial cells. *J Pharmacol Exp Ther* 288:1357-66.

Wallace, J. M., R. Lim, B. L. Browdy, P. C. Hopewell, J. Glassroth, M. J. Rosen, L. B. Reichman, and P. A. Kvale.1998. Risk factors and outcomes associated with identification of *Aspergillus* in respiratory specimens from persons with HIV disease. Pulmonary complications of HIV infection study group. *Chest* 114(1):131-7.

Whitfield, R. M., L. M. Bechtel, and G. H. Starich. 1997. The impact of ethanol and Marinol/marijuana usage on HIV+/AIDS patients undergoing azidothymidine, azidothymidine/dideoxycytidine, or dideoxyinosine therapy. *Alcohol Clin Exp Res* 21(1): 122-7.

Wing, D. R., J. T. A. Leuschner, G. A. Brent, D. J. Harvey, and W. D. M. Paton. 1985. Quantification of *in vivo* membrane associated delta-9-tetrahydrocannabinol and its effects on membrane fluidity. *Proceedings of the 9th International Congress of Pharmacology 3rd satellite symposium on cannabis*. Harvey, D. J. Oxford: IRL Press.

Zhu, L. X., S. Sharma, M. Stolina, B. Gardner, M. D. Roth, D. P. Tashkin, and S. M. Dubinett. 2000. Delta-9-tetrahydrocannabinol inhibits antitumor immunity by a CB2 receptor-mediated, cytokine-dependent pathway. *J Immunol* 165(1):373-80.

Zimmerman, S., A. M. Zimmerman, I. L. Cameron, and H. L. Lawrence. 1977. Delta1-tetrahydrocannabinol, cannabidiol and cannabinol effects on the immune response of mice. *Pharmacology* 15:10-23.

Effects of Smoked Marijuana on the Lung and Its Immune Defenses: Implications for Medicinal Use in HIV-Infected Patients

Donald P. Tashkin

SUMMARY. Habitual marijuana smoking may cause a number of potentially harmful effects on the lung, including the following: (1) acute and chronic bronchitis; (2) extensive histopathologic alterations in the cells lining the bronchial passages that could impair mucociliary clearance or predispose to malignancy; (3) increased accumulation of inflammatory cells (alveolar macrophages) in the lung; and (4) impairment in the function of these important immune-effector cells, including their ability to kill microorganisms and to produce protective pro-inflammatory cytokines. The major potential pulmonary consequences of habitual marijuana use are pulmonary infection and respiratory cancer. Infectious complications could be due to smoking-related damage to the mucociliary clearance mechanism, marijuana-related impairment in the antimicrobial function of alveolar macrophages and/or fungal or bacterial contamination of marijuana. Patients with pre-existing immune deficits

Donald P. Tashkin, MD, is affiliated with the Division of Pulmonary and Critical Care Medicine, UCLA School of Medicine.

Address correspondence to: Donald P. Tashkin, MD, Professor of Medicine, Department of Medicine, UCLA School of Medicine, 10833 Le Conte Avenue, Los Angeles, CA 90095-1690 (E-mail: dtashkin@mednet.ucla.edu).

Supported by U.S. Public Health Service Grant (National Institute on Drug Abuse) No. R37 DA-03018.

[Haworth co-indexing entry note]: "Effects of Smoked Marijuana on the Lung and Its Immune Defenses: Implications for Medicinal Use in HIV-Infected Patients." Tashkin, Donald P. Co-published simultaneously in *Journal of Cannabis Therapeutics* (The Haworth Integrative Healing Press, an imprint of The Haworth Press, Inc.) Vol. 1, No. 3/4, 2001, pp. 87-102; and: *Cannabis Therapeutics in HIV/AIDS* (ed: Ethan Russo) The Haworth Integrative Healing Press, an imprint of The Haworth Press, Inc., 2001, pp. 87-102. Single or multiple copies of this article are available for a fee from The Haworth Document Delivery Service [1-800-342-9678, 9:00 a.m. - 5:00 p.m. (EST). E-mail address: getinfo@haworthpressinc.com].

due to AIDS could be particularly susceptible to pulmonary infectious complications of marijuana use. *[Article copies available for a fee from The Haworth Document Delivery Service: 1-800-342-9678. E-mail address: <getinfo@haworthpressinc.com> Website: <http://www.HaworthPress.com> © 2001 by The Haworth Press, Inc. All rights reserved.]*

KEYWORDS. Pulmonary function, cannabis, medical marijuana, HIV, AIDS

INTRODUCTION

In view of the continuing interest in the medical application of marijuana for treatment of AIDS-related symptoms, it is important to re-examine the effects of marijuana smoking on the lung and its biologic defenses against infection. This issue is of practical importance in assessing the risk-benefit ratio of cannabis therapy in the immune-suppressed patient, i.e., the relative risk of pneumonia and other potential, serious infectious complications of marijuana in relation to its possible benefits in stimulating appetite, combating nausea, relieving pain, etc. The present review will focus mainly on human observational and epidemiological studies conducted within the past two decades pertaining to the impact of marijuana smoking on lung structure and function and on respiratory illness. The reader is referred to a recent review article that also addresses the airway effects of illicit smoked substances (Tashkin 2001).

EFFECTS ON RESPIRATORY SYMPTOMS

Three separate community-based studies reported within the past 15 years have shown that habitual daily or near-daily use of marijuana is associated with both chronic and acute respiratory symptoms, indicative of chronic and acute bronchitis.

In a Los Angeles-based convenience sample of 144 daily smokers of marijuana only (MS, mean age 32 yrs), 135 smokers of both marijuana and tobacco (MTS, mean age 34 yrs), 70 smokers of tobacco only (TS, mean age 37 yrs) and 97 nonsmokers (NS, mean age 32 yrs), MS had a significantly higher prevalence than NS ($P < 0.05$) of chronic cough (18% vs. 0%, respectively), chronic sputum production (20% vs. 0%), wheeze (25% vs. 3.5%) and episodes of acute bronchitis (13% vs. 2%) (Tashkin et al. 1987). Chronic cough was defined as cough on most days for at least three months a year for two or more consecutive years and conforms to the accepted definition of "chronic bronchitis" (American Thoracic Society 1987). In contrast, the prevalence of symptoms of chronic and acute bronchitis did not differ significantly between MS and TS, and no additive effects of marijuana and tobacco were found.

In a parallel Tucson-based study of young (mean 27 yrs) MS (n = 54), MTS (n = 56), TS (n = 20) and NS (n = 502) recruited from a random stratified cluster of households in the community, significantly more MS than NS reported cough, sputum, wheeze and shortness of breath (p $\leq$ 0.05) (Bloom et al. 1987). Moreover, an additive effect of marijuana and tobacco on chronic respiratory symptoms was noted, in contrast to the findings from the Los Angeles study (Tashkin et al. 1987).

In a more recent study of 91 cannabis-dependent subjects selected from a total of 943 young adults 21 yrs of age who comprised a birth cohort born in Dunedin, New Zealand, respiratory symptoms were significantly more frequent in cannabis-dependent, nonsmokers of tobacco compared to non-tobacco smoking controls, including early morning sputum production (144% higher prevalence); wheezing apart from colds (61%); exertional dyspnea (65%); and night-time awakenings with chest tightness (72%) (Taylor et al. 2000). Interestingly, the prevalence of respiratory symptoms in cannabis-dependent subjects was similar to that in smokers of $\leq$ 1/2 pack of tobacco cigarettes/day.

EFFECTS ON LUNG FUNCTION

Findings from the three community-based studies of the pulmonary status of regular marijuana users cited above have revealed conflicting effects of habitual marijuana use on lung function. In the Tucson study, MS, compared to NS, showed significantly lower values for the ratio of forced expired volume in one second (FEV_1) to forced vital capacity (FVC), a sensitive and specific indicator of airflow obstruction (Bloom et al. 1987). Even lower values for FEV_1/FVC ratio were observed in MS than TS, although the mean values for this measure were still within statistically normal limits. From these observations the authors concluded that regular marijuana smoking among young individuals may be an important risk factor for the subsequent development of obstructive airways disease. A follow-up study of the same cohort demonstrated a significant reduction in FEV_1 and FEV_1/FVC ratio in relation to previous use of marijuana, a finding that was interpreted as suggesting that continuing marijuana smoking may lead to a progressive decline in lung function (Sherrill et al. 1991).

In the more recent study from New Zealand, 36% of 21-yr-old cannabis-dependent subjects (two-thirds of whom had developed cannabis dependence since age 18), demonstrated a reduced FEV_1/FVC ratio (< 0.80), compared to only 20% of the nonsmokers from the same birth cohort (p = 0.04) (Taylor et al. 2000). The authors concluded that only a relatively short duration of heavy cannabis use can lead to early airways obstruction in young individuals. It is not clear, however, whether adequate adjustment was made for the possible confounding of these findings by concomitant tobacco use.

The above findings are not supported by the results of the Los Angeles study of 124 MS, 56 TS, 113 MTS and 92 NS (Tashkin et al. 1987). In the latter study, no association was observed between heavy, habitual use of marijuana (mean of > 3 joints/day for > 15 yrs) and abnormalities not only in FEV_1 or FEV_1/FVC ratio, but also in even more sensitive measures of early obstructive ventilatory impairment, including forced expiratory flow rates at low lung volumes and indices derived from single-breath nitrogen washout. Abnormalities in the latter tests are commonly found in tobacco cigarette smokers, some of who are destined to develop clinically significant chronic obstructive pulmonary disease. In addition, regular use of marijuana was not associated with any abnormality in the single-breath diffusing capacity for carbon monoxide (D_LCO), a sensitive physiologic indicator of emphysema (Tashkin et al. 1987). On the other hand, regular tobacco smoking was associated with abnormalities in most of the tests of airways function, as well as in D_LCO, and heavy habitual marijuana use did not potentiate any of the adverse effects of concomitant tobacco smoking on lung function in dual smokers of marijuana and tobacco.

More recently, the Los Angeles investigators sought to determine whether regular marijuana smoking might lead to a progressive decline in lung function with age and continuing smoking that was not evident in the earlier analysis of the cross-sectional data for lung function (Tashkin et al. 1997). They measured FEV_1 sequentially at intervals of ≥ 1 yr for up to 8 yrs in 87 MS, 42 TS, 63 MTS and 63 NS. While they noted that tobacco smoking was associated with a significant age-related decline in FEV_1 compared to the change in NS, they were unable to detect an effect of even heavy marijuana smoking (3 joints/d) on FEV_1 decline, nor did they observe any additive effect of marijuana and tobacco. Since chronic obstructive pulmonary disease (chronic obstructive bronchitis and/or emphysema) is characterized by an excessive age-related decline in FEV_1, these findings argue against an association between regular marijuana smoking and the development of chronic obstructive pulmonary disease. This conclusion is supported by the results of earlier studies in rats exposed to progressively increasing doses of marijuana or tobacco smoke for six months in which the lungs of the tobacco-exposed rats, but *not* those of the marijuana-exposed rats or the unexposed control animals, showed anatomic and physiologic evidence of emphysema (Huber and Mahajan 1988).

EFFECTS ON AIRWAY PATHOLOGY

It is possible that habitual cannabis smoking may cause airway injury and inflammation in the absence of either respiratory symptoms or any demonstrable alteration in lung function. Therefore, to determine the effects of marijuana and tobacco smoking on the gross appearance of the visible portion of the lower respiratory tract of healthy individuals, Roth et al. (1998) performed videobronchoscopy on a small cohort of 40 relatively asymptomatic nonsmokers (NS; n = 10), smokers of marijuana only (MS; n = 10), smokers of tobacco only (TS; n = 10) and smokers of both marijuana and tobacco (MTS; n = 10), all of whom had no or few abnormalities in lung function. A visual bronchitis index score was used to evaluate the presence and extent of airway erythema (redness), edema (swelling) and hypersecretion. Biopsies of the bronchial mucosa were also performed to correlate the visual endoscopic observations with microscopic histopathologic evidence of airway injury and inflammation (vascular hyperplasia, submucosal edema, inflammatory cell infiltrates and hyperplasia of surface mucus-secreting [goblet] cells). In addition, bronchial lavage (saline rinse) was performed to evaluate the peripheral airways for evidence of inflammation (reflected by increased numbers of neutrophils) and/or elevations in interleukin-8 (IL-8), a potent neutrophil chemoattractant and activator. Bronchitis index scores were found to be significantly higher in MS, TS and MTS than in NS. Bronchial mucosal biopsies were positive for two of the histopathologic features of airway injury in 97% of all smokers and for three criteria in 72%, whereas none of the biopsies from NS showed greater than one positive finding. The percentage of neutrophils in bronchial lavage fluid correlated with IL-8 levels and exceeded 20% in 0 of 10 NS, 1 of 9 MS, 2 of 9 TS, and 5 of 10 MTS. These findings suggest that regular smoking of marijuana and/or tobacco by young adults is associated with a high frequency of endoscopically and microscopically apparent airway injury and inflammation even in the absence of any symptoms or physiologic evidence of injury.

The effect of habitual use of marijuana on the microscopic pathology of the lower airways was systematically evaluated by a single "blinded" pathologist from bronchial mucosal biopsies obtained at bronchoscopy from healthy volunteer subjects participating in the Los Angeles cohort study (Fligiel et al. 1997). These subjects included 40 MS, 31 TS, 44 MTS and 53 NS, most of who did not report significant respiratory symptoms or demonstrate significant abnormalities in lung function. The histopathologic features that were examined included basal cell hyperplasia; stratification; squamous metaplasia; goblet cell hyperplasia; cellular disorganization; nuclear variation; mitotic figures; increased nuclear-to-cytoplasmic ratio; inflammation; and basement membrane thickening. Regular smoking of marijuana alone (average of 3-4 joints per day) was associated with a greater frequency and severity of abnormalities for most of the features examined compared to the changes noted in the nonsmokers and at least as extensive abnormalities as those found in the smokers of tobacco alone (22 cigarettes per day). The similar frequency and extent of bronchial histopathology in the marijuana-only compared to the tobacco-only smokers is noteworthy in view of the marked disparity between the daily number of marijuana vs. tobacco cigarettes consumed by these two groups of subjects. Interestingly, for nearly all histological features examined, abnormalities were noted more commonly in the combined smokers of marijuana plus tobacco than in smokers of either substance alone, implying additive effects of the two smoked substances on airway injury.

These findings have the following important implications:

- Habitual marijuana smoking can cause potentially serious airway pathology at a relatively early age even in the absence of any clinical or physiologic evidence of disease.
- Regular marijuana use produces at least as much damage to the mucosa of the larger airways as the regular smoking of tobacco, despite the considerably smaller daily number of marijuana joints smoked by the MS (average of 3-4 joints/d) than the daily number of tobacco cigarettes smoked by the TS (mean of 22 cigarettes/d), suggesting that marijuana has a more damaging effect than tobacco per cigarette smoked. The similarity in airway histopathology despite the disparity in the amount of plant substance smoked might be explained, at least partly, by the four-fold increase in deposition of tar from a single marijuana cigarette compared to a tobacco cigarette of the same weight (Wu et al. 1988). The latter increase in deposition could be due to differences in cigarette filtration and smoking technique for the two types of cigarettes: marijuana cigarettes do not have filter tips, are more loosely packed and are generally smoked with a four-fold longer breathholding time than tobacco cigarettes. The differences in filtration enhance delivery of tar to the smoker's mouth from marijuana compared to tobacco cigarettes, and the far longer breathholding time employed in smoking marijuana than tobacco provides more opportunity for respiratory deposition of ultra-fine smoke particulates and absorption of toxic gas-phase constituents in the smoke (Wu et al. 1988; Tashkin et al. 1991).
- The observation that marijuana and tobacco appear to have additive effects on bronchial epithelial histopathology in the combined smokers of both substances is of concern since the prevalence of tobacco smoking is substantially higher among marijuana smokers than nonsmokers of marijuana. For example, in the UCLA cohort, approximately 50% of the marijuana smokers also smoked tobacco, whereas the prevalence of tobacco smoking among adults in California in general is approximately 20%.
- Some of the histopathologic changes in the marijuana smokers, notably the frequent loss of ciliated bronchial epithelial cells and their replacement by non-ciliated cells, such as hyperplastic mucus-secreting (goblet)

cells or reserve (basal) cells, or by metaplastic squamous epithelium, could explain the high frequency of symptoms of chronic bronchitis (chronic cough and sputum production) in smokers of marijuana alone. The hair-like projections (cilia) of the normal ciliated bronchial epithelial cells play an important role in mucociliary clearance of secretions. Excessive mucus production by hyperplastic goblet cells (and by hypertrophied submucosal mucus glands) and diminished clearance of these secretions because of the loss of cilia can lead to an accumulation of excess mucus, leaving cough as the only mechanism for mucus clearance. Since the mucus lining the airways also traps inhaled bacteria, other microorganisms and other potentially harmful particles, an intact mucociliary clearance mechanism is the lung's first line of defense against infection and other noxious insults. Marijuana-related damage to this mechanism could therefore predispose to lower respiratory tract infection and other adverse consequences of inhaled particulates.

• A carcinogenic effect of marijuana is suggested by certain histopathologic alterations in the bronchial epithelium of smokers of marijuana with or without tobacco. These include squamous metaplasia, cellular disorganization, nuclear variation, mitotic figures and increased nuclear-to-cytoplasmic ratio, which have long been considered to represent potential precursors for the subsequent development of bronchogenic carcinoma (Auerbach et al. 1961).

BRONCHIAL EXPRESSION OF IMMUNOHISTOCHEMICAL MARKERS OF DYSREGULATED GROWTH AND PRE-TUMOR PROGRESSION

A number of genetic alterations are responsible for the transformation of lung cells from normal to cancerous. Bronchial biopsies obtained in 12 MS, 14 TS, 9 MTS and 28 MTS from the UCLA cohort were therefore examined for alterations in some of the genes involved in the pathogenesis of lung cancer, as reflected by surrogate end-point markers that have been linked to an increased risk of lung cancer. Immunohistological studies of these biopsies showed marked overexpression in the bronchial epithelium of MS of Ki-67 (a marker of cell proliferation) and epidermal growth factor receptor (EGFR) (Barsky et al. 1998). Moreover, p53, one of the most common tumor suppressor genes altered in human cancers, was expressed in 11% of subjects who smoked marijuana together with tobacco. These findings suggest that smoking marijuana, like tobacco smoking, causes dysregulated growth of bronchial epithelial cells, possibly reflecting an increased risk of marijuana smokers for the subsequent development of lung cancer.

EFFECTS ON ALVEOLAR MACROPHAGES

Effects on Alveolar Macrophage Structure

Alveolar macrophages (AMs) are the major cells that reside in the peripheral air spaces of the lung and normally constitute over 90% of the cells recovered by bronchoalveolar lavage (BAL). These important immune effector cells play a crucial role in the lung's immune defense system. MS, TS and MTS all show an increase in the number of AMs recovered from the distal air spaces by BAL, compared to NS in the order of MTS > TS > MS > NS, and the effects of marijuana and tobacco smoking on the accumulation of AMs in the lung appear additive (Barbers et al. 1987). Examination of the ultrastructure of AMs recovered by BAL from smokers of marijuana and/or tobacco and nonsmokers by transmission electron microscopy has revealed marked abnormalities in the AMs of the smokers of either or both substances, consisting mainly of larger and more complex cytoplasmic inclusions than observed in the AMs of nonsmokers (Beals et al. 1989). Furthermore, ultrastructural differences were noted between the AMs of MS and TS, suggesting that exposure to marijuana or tobacco could lead to differences in the functional activity of these cells.

Effects on Alveolar Macrophage Function

The functional activity of human alveolar macrophages has been assessed by examination of their microbicidal activity and their production of reactive oxygen species, reactive nitrogen intermediates and inflammatory cytokines.

MICROBICIDAL ACTIVITY

AMs from both MS and TS have been shown to be impaired in their ability to kill *Candida albicans* (Sherman et al. 1991a) and *Candida pseudotropicalis* (Baldwin et al. 1997) compared to AMs from NS, although no defect in phagocytosis for fungi was noted (Sherman et al. 1991a). AMs from MS, but not those from TS, have also been shown to be deficient in their ability both to phagocytose and to kill the pathogenic bacterium, *Staphylococcus aureus*. The cause of these marijuana-related deficits in AM fungicidal activity and bacterial phagocytosis and killing is unclear but could be due, at least partly, to marijuana-induced deficiencies in the production of toxic oxygen species or reactive nitrogen intermediates, such as nitric oxide.

PRODUCTION OF REACTIVE OXYGEN SPECIES
("RESPIRATORY BURST")

Earlier studies demonstrated a reduced ability of AMs from MS to generate superoxide anion (O_2) both under basal conditions (compared to AMs from either NS or TS) and when stimulated (compared to AMs from TS), in contrast to an enhanced generation of O_2^- by AMs from TS under both basal and respiratory-burst stimulated conditions (Sherman et al. 1991a,b). Since reactive oxygen species serve as important effector molecules for microbial killing, the different respiratory burst characteristics of AMs from MS compared to those of AMs obtained from TS imply that different mechanisms may contribute to impairment of fungicidal activity of alveolar macrophages derived from smokers of these two different substances. It is tempting to speculate, however, that, since oxidants, including O_2^-, released from AMs, can also cause lung tissue injury, the marijuana-related impairment in the respiratory burst activity of AMs may provide protection against smoke-related damage to the peripheral airways and alveoli. Thus, it is possible that the dampening effect of marijuana smoking on the production of toxic oxygen radicals by immune effector cells in the lung could account for the absence of abnormalities in small airways function and alveolar diffusing capacity (physiologic markers of tobacco-related small airways disease and/or emphysema) in smokers of marijuana alone, in contrast to the presence of such physiologic abnormalities in smokers of tobacco, with or without marijuana (Sherman et al. 1991a,b).

PRODUCTION OF REACTIVE NITROGEN INTERMEDIATES
AND PRO-INFLAMMATORY CYTOKINES

Preliminary data suggest that the impairment in the bactericidal activity of AMs from MS may be due to a marijuana-related impairment in production of reactive nitrogen intermediates (e.g., nitric oxide), which also serve as important effector molecules in bacterial killing. This impairment, in turn, could be secondary to a marijuana-related inhibition of AM production of inducible nitric oxide synthase (iNOS) in the course of infection (Baldwin et al. 2000). *In vitro* studies using AMs from MS in killing assays for *S. aureus* in the presence or absence of an inhibitor of iNOS with and without the addition of specific pro-inflammatory cytokines (interferon-γ [INFγ] and granulocyte-macrophage colony stimulating factor [GM-CSF]) suggest that the inhibition in bactericidal activity may be due to a marijuana-related impairment in production of key cytokines (e.g., INFγ and GM-CSF) that mediate the induction of iNOS. Other data indicating an inhibition of lipopolysaccharide-stimulated production of TNF-α, IL-6 and GM-CSF by AMs from MS but not from TS provide further support for this hypothesis (Baldwin et al. 1997).

EFFECTS ON OTHER IMMUNE CELLS

Several *in vitro* and animal studies suggest that Δ^9-tetrahydrocannabinol (THC) is a powerful immune modulator and that it has a predominantly immunosuppressive effect on a variety of immune cells, including macrophages, natural killer cells and T lymphocytes (Klein, Friedman and Specter 1998). These observations are consistent with the finding of cannabinoid (CB) receptors on immune cells (Bouaboula et al. 1993). The immunosuppressive effect of THC appears to be due to its inhibition of lymphocyte production of immunostimulatory helper T cell type-1 cytokines (e.g., interleukin-2 [IL-2] and interferon gamma [IFN-γ]) and its parallel promotion of the production of immunoinhibitory helper T cell type-2 cytokines, such as interleukin-10 [IL-10] and interleukin-4 [IL-4] (Newton, 1994). It is possible that this immunosuppressive effect of THC could impair the host's ability to develop an antibacterial immune response and thereby facilitate bacterial infection. This possibility was studied in a mouse model of *Legionella pneumophila,* a cause of community-acquired and opportunistic pneumonia (Newton, Klein and Friedman 1994). Mice pre-treated with Δ^9-THC prior to infection with a sublethal dose of *L. pneumophila* failed to develop cell-mediated protective immunity and died when re-challenged with the organism, while control mice not pre-treated with Δ^9-THC became immune to repeated infection and survived. It is possible that a similar mechanism could be responsible for an increased predisposition of human users of marijuana to pulmonary infection.

CLINICAL IMPLICATIONS

The clinical implications of the above findings concerning the impact of regular marijuana smoking on the microbicidal activity of human AMs, as well as the inhibitory effect of THC on the ability of experimental animals to develop a protective anti-bacterial immune response, are that marijuana smoking may impair the lung's defense against infection, in part due to impairment in the critical antimicrobial function of alveolar macrophages, thus predisposing to pneumonia. The associated impairment in tracheobronchial mucociliary function (implied by the histopathologic evidence of marijuana-associated damage to the normal ciliated epithelial lining of the lower respiratory tract) further undermines the ability of the lung to defend itself against infections. In marijuana smokers with HIV infection, the combined effects of these two factors could add to the already increased risk of immunosuppressed patients with AIDS for pulmonary infection. The reported frequent contamination of marijuana with the fungus, *Aspergillus fumigatus,* (Kagen et al. 1983) and with potentially pathogenic gram-negative bacteria (Ungerleider et al. 1982) could further heighten the risk of opportunistic fungal and bacterial pneumonia in the immunocompromised patient. A few clinical case reports and limited epidemiological studies (*vide infra*) provide some clues, but as yet no definitive evidence, as to the real risks of immunocompromised patients for the development or respiratory infection as a complication of marijuana smoking.

CLINICAL CASE REPORTS

Several clinical cases have been reported of invasive *Aspergillus* pneumonia in immunocompromised patients, including patients with AIDS (Denning et al. 1991), chronic granulomatous disease (Chusid et al. 1975), bone marrow transplantation (Hamadeh et al. 1988), renal transplantation (Marks et al. 1996) or small cell lung cancer treated with chemotherapy (Sutton, Lum, and Torti 1986), all of whom smoked marijuana. The precise role of marijuana in these cases of invasive pulmonary aspergillosis is unclear. While it is possible that the opportunistic fungal pulmonary infection in these patients may have been due primarily to their underlying immune compromise in the face of possible contamination of marijuana with *Aspergillus* (Kagen et al. 1983), the further possibility that an independent superimposed effect of marijuana smoking on pulmonary host defenses was a critical factor cannot be excluded. It is also possible that habitual marijuana smokers without any identifiable underlying immune deficiency could be predisposed to pulmonary infection as a consequence of the deficits in the lung's host defense caused by regular cannabis use. Recently, a 23-yr-old heavy smoker of both marijuana and tobacco with a history of intravenous opioid use but no clinical evidence of an underlying immune deficiency was reported to have developed miliary necrotizing granulomata, associated with progressive exertional dyspnea, bilateral nodular pulmonary infiltrates and a blackened alveolar exudate of carbon-laded macrophages (Cunningham et al. 2000). Although actual fungal infection was not documented, the authors suspected either infection with an unidentified fungus inhaled with the marijuana smoke or hypersensitivity to inhaled fungi as the most likely cause of the necrotizing granulomata.

EPIDEMIOLOGICAL STUDIES

Outpatient Visits for Respiratory Illness

In an epidemiological cohort study of the impact of marijuana smoking on the health care utilization of Kaiser Permanente health plan members, marijuana smoking history was ascertained from a comprehensive, multi-phasic health screening questionnaire and the medical experience of daily or near-daily users of marijuana who never smoked tobacco (n = 452), as ascertained from medical records reviews, was compared with that of a demographically similar group of nonsmokers of either substance (n = 450) (Polen et al. 1993). Frequent marijuana smokers had small but significantly increased risks of outpatient visits for respiratory illness (relative risk [RR] = 1.19; 95% C.I. = 1.02, 1.16), as well as for other types of illness, compared with nonsmokers, in addition to a small increased risk of hospitalization. Neither independent nor additive or interactive effects of tobacco combined with marijuana were examined in this study.

Studies in Subjects with AIDS or HIV-Seropositivity

In an early, small-scale case-control study of 31 patients with severe manifestations of AIDS (13 with confirmed Kaposi's sarcoma and 18 with an opportunistic infection) compared with 29 symptom-free patients referred with possible AIDS, marijuana use was associated with a significantly increased risk for progression to Kaposi's sarcoma or opportunistic infection (OR = 3.7 [95% C.I. 1.10-12.30]; p < 0.05) (Newell et al. 1985). In another early prospective study in which logistic regression was used to assess lifestyle factors associated with progression or non-progression of 386 HIV seropositive individuals to end-stage AIDS within 2-3 years of enrollment, marijuana use in the preceding 3 months was identified as one of only two lifestyle factors or the only factor associated with progression to AIDS (n = 32) in univariate or multivariate analyses, respectively (Tindall et al. 1988). A more recent cohort study of risk factors for the first episode of bacterial pneumonia in 629 HIV-seropositive injection drug users (IDUs), of whom 40 subsequently developed pneumonia, revealed that smoking illicit substances (marijuana or crack cocaine) was significantly associated with the development of bacterial pneumonia in multivariate analysis (OR = 2.24; 95% C.I. 1.03-4.89) (Caiaffa et al. 1994). It is particularly noteworthy that among HIV-seropositive IDUs with a previous history of *Pneumocystis carinii* pneumonia, smoking illicit drugs had the strongest effect on risk of bacterial pneumonia (OR = 22.94; 95% C.I. 2.18-241.10). These few epidemiological studies suggest that HIV-seropositive patients who smoke marijuana regularly may be particularly vulnerable to opportunistic pulmonary infection. However, the possible incrimination of marijuana smoking for predisposing HIV-seropositive patients to pneumonia requires further investigation by more rigorous epidemiological studies, particularly in view of the growing interest in medicinal marijuana for patients with AIDS.

Mortality

The relationship of marijuana use to mortality was examined in a cohort of 65,171 Kaiser Permanente health care members, 15-49 yrs of age, who completed health-screening questionnaires that included questions on marijuana use (Sidney et al. 1997). Follow-up for assessing mortality was conducted for 6-12 yrs following questionnaire completion. Current marijuana use was not associated with a significantly higher risk of mortality in either men or women, compared with nonuse, except for an increased risk of death due to AIDS in men. However, the latter association was felt to be due to confounding by male homosexual behavior among the current marijuana smokers, rather than an effect of marijuana itself on mortality due to AIDS.

OTHER CLINICAL CONSEQUENCES

Barotrauma and Lung Bullae

Isolated cases of spontaneous pneumothorax and/or pneumomediastinum have been temporally associated with marijuana use (Feldman et al. 1993; Mattox 1976; Miller. Spiekerman and Hepper 1972). These complications are believed to involve barotrauma to the lung from the increased intrathoracic pressure that develops when a marijuana smoker performs a Valsalva maneuver against a closed glottis after deep inhalation of the smoke in an effort to "pressurize" the smoke within the lung to enhance absorption of THC. Several cases of large upper zone lung bullae have recently been reported in otherwise healthy young male marijuana smokers with relatively little exposure to tobacco (Johnson et al. 2000) The mechanism for bulla formation in these cases could be due to a direct toxic effect of components in marijuana smoke on the lungs of susceptible smokers and/or airway barotrauma related to the high intrathoracic pressures generated during marijuana smoking. The clinical significance of pneumothorax and/or pneumomediastinum could be exaggerated in patients with AIDS who already have pulmonary deficits due to effects of current or previous pulmonary infectious or noninfectious pulmonary complications of AIDS.

CONCLUSION

Frequent marijuana use can cause airway injury, lung inflammation and impaired pulmonary defense against infection. The major potential pulmonary consequence of habitual marijuana use of particular relevance to patients with AIDS is superimposed pulmonary infection, which could be life threatening in the seriously immunocompromised patient. In view of the immunosuppressive effect of THC, the possibility that regular marijuana use could enhance progression of HIV infection itself needs to be considered, although this possibility remains unexplored to date. A few mainly older epidemiological studies in

HIV-positive individuals have identified marijuana use as a significant risk factor for acquisition of opportunistic infections and/or Kaposi's sarcoma. Further investigation of the real risks of pulmonary complications from regular marijuana use by HIV-positive patients is required using rigorous epidemiological methodology.

REFERENCES

American Thoracic Society. 1987. Standards for the diagnosis and care of patients with chronic obstructive pulmonary disease (COPD) and asthma. *Am Rev Respir Dis* 136:229-243.

Auerbach, O., A.P. Stout, E.C. Hammond, and L. Garfinkel. 1962. Changes in bronchial epithelium in relation to sex, age, residence, smoking and pneumonia. *N Engl J Med* 267:111-119.

Baldwin, G.C., D.P. Tashkin, D.M. Buckley, A.N. Park, D.M. Dubinett, and M.D. Roth. 1997. Habitual smoking of marijuana and cocaine impairs alveolar macrophage function and cytokine production. *J Respir Crit Care Med* 156:1606-1613.

Baldwin, G.C., R. Choi, A.H. Shey, E.C. Kleerup, M.D. Roth, and D.P. Tashkin. 2000. Nitric oxide: A mediator of alveolar macrophage antimicrobial activity compromised in cocaine and marijuana smokers. *Am J Respir Crit Care Med* 161: A124.

Barbers, R.G., H. Gong, Jr, D.P. Tashkin, J. Oishi, and J.M. Wallace: Differential examination of bronchoalveolar lavage cells in tobacco cigarette and marijuana smokers. *Am Rev Respir Dis* 135:1271-1275.

Barsky, S.H., M.D. Roth, E.C. Kleerup, M. Simmons, and D.P. Tashkin. 1998. Similar molecular alterations in bronchial epithelium are observed in habitual smokers of marijuana, cocaine and/or tobacco. *J Natl Canc Inst* 90:1198-1204.

Beals, T.F., S.E.G. Fligiel, S. Stuth, and D.P. Tashkin. 1989. Morphological alterations of alveolar macrophages from marijuana smokers. *Am Rev Respir Dis* 139 (part 2):A336.

Bloom, J.W., W.T. Kaltenborn, P. Paoletti, A. Camilli, M.D. Lebowitz. 1987. Respiratory effects of on-tobacco cigarettes. *Brit Med J* 295:1516-1518.

Bouaboula, M, M. Rinaldi, P. Carayon, C. Carillon, B. Delpech, D. Shire, G. Le Fur, and P. Casellas. 1993. Cannabinoid-receptor expression in human leukocytes. *Eur J Biochem* 214:173-80.

Caiaffa, W.T., D. Vlahov, N.M. Graham, J. Astemborski, L. Solomon, K.E. Nelson, and A. Nelson. 1994. Drug smoking, *Pneumocystis carinii* pneumonia, and immunosuppression increase risk of bacterial pneumonia in human immunodeficiency virus-seropositive infection drug users. *Am Rev Respir Dis* 150:1493-98.

Chusid, M.J., J.A. Gelfland, C. Nutter, A.S. Fauci. 1975. Pulmonary aspergillosis, inhalation of contaminated marijuana smoke, chronic granulomatous disease. *Ann Intern Med* 82:682-683.

Cunnington, D., H. Teichtahl, J.M. Hunt, C. Dow, and R. Valentine. 2000. Necrotizing pulmonary granulomata in a marijuana smoker. *Chest* 117:1511-1514.

Denning, D.W., S.E. Follansbee, M. Scolaro, S. Norris, H. Edelstein, and D.A. Stevens. 1991. Pulmonary aspergillosis in the acquired immunodeficiency syndrome. *N Engl J Med* 324:654-662.

Feldman, A.L., J.T. Sullivan, M.A. Passero, and D.C. Lewis. 1993. Pneumothorax in polysubstance abusing marijuana and tobacco smokers: 3 cases. *J Substance Abuse* 5:183-186.

Fligiel, S.E.G., M.D. Roth, E.C. Kleerup, S.H. Barsky, M.S. Simmons, and D.P. Tashkin. 1997. Tracheobronchial histopathology in habitual smokers of cocaine, marijuana and/or tobacco. *Chest* 112:319-326.

Hamadeh, R., A. Ardehali, R.M. Locksley, and M.K. York. 1988. Fatal aspergillosis associated with smoking contaminated marijuana in a marrow transplant recipient. *Chest* 94:432-433.

Huber, G.L., and V.K. Mahajan. 1987. The comparative response of the lung to marihuana or tobacco smoke inhalation. In G. Chesher, P. Consroe & R. Musty (Eds.), *Marijuana: An International Research Report. Proceedings of Melbourne Symposium on Cannabis 2-4 September*. (National Campaign Against Drug Abuse Monograph Series No. 7, pp. 19-24). Canberra: Australian Government Publishing Service.

Johnson, M.K., R.P. Smith, D. Morrison, G. Laszlo, and R.J. White. 2000. Large lung bullae in marijuana smokers. *Thorax* 55:340-342.

Kagen, S.L., V.P. Kurup, P.C. Sohnle, and J.N. Fink. 1983. Marijuana smoking and fungal sensitization. *J Allergy Clin Immunol* 71:389-393.

Klein, T.W., H. Friedman, and S. Specter. 1998. Marijuana, immunity and infection. *J Neuroimmunol* 83:102-115, 1998.

Marks, W.H., L. Florence, J. Lieberman, P. Chapman, D. Howard, P. Roberts, and D. Perkinson. 1996. Successfully treated invasive pulmonary aspergillosis associated with smoking marijuana in a renal transplant recipient. *Transplantation* 61:1771-1783.

Mattox, K.L. 1976. Pneumomediastinum in heroin and marijuana users. *J Amer Coll Emerg Phys* 5:26-28.

Miller, W.E., R.E. Spiekerman, and N.G. Hepper. 1972. Pneumomediastinum resulting from performing Valsalva maneuvers during marijuana smoking. *Chest* 62: 233-234

Newell, G.R., P.W. Mansell, M.B. Wilson, H.K. Lynch, M.R. Spitz, and E.M. Hersh. 1985. Risk factor analysis among men referred for possible acquired immune deficiency syndrome. *Prevent Med* 14:81-91.

Newton, C.A., T.W. Klein, and H. Friedman. 1994. Secondary immunity to *Legionella pneumophila* and Th1 activity are suppressed by Δ^9-tetrahydrocannabinol injection. *Infect Immun* 62:4015-4020.

Polen, M.R., S. Sidney, I.S. Tekawa, M. Sadler, G.D. Friedmean. 1993. Health care use by frequent marijuana smokers who do not smoke tobacco. *West J Med* 158: 596-601.

Roth, M.D., A. Arora, S.H. Barsky, E.C. Kleerup, M. Simmons, and D.P. Tashkin. 1998. Visual and pathologic evidence of injury to the airways of young marijuana smokers. *Am J Respir Crit Care Med* 157:928-937.

Sherman, M.P., L.A. Campbell, H. Gong, Jr., M.D. Roth, and D.P. Tashkin. 1991. Respiratory burst and microbicidal characteristics of pulmonary alveolar macrophages recovered from smokers of marijuana alone, smokers of tobacco alone, smokers of marijuana and tobacco and nonsmokers. *Am Rev Respir Dis* 144:1351-1356.

Sherman, M.P., M.D. Roth, H. Gong, Jr., and D.P. Tashkin. 1991a. Marijuana smoking, pulmonary function and lung macrophage oxidant release. *Pharmacol Biochem Behav* 40:663-669.

Sherrill, D.L., M. Krzyzanowski, J.W. Bloom, M.D. Lebowitz. 1991b. Respiratory effects of non-tobacco cigarettes: A longitudinal study in general population. *Internat J Epidem* 20:132-137.

Sidney, S., Beck, J.E., I.S. Tekawa, C.P. Quesenberry, Jr., and G.D. Friedman. 1997. Marijuana use and mortality. *Am J Public Health* 87:585:590.

Sutton, S., B.L. Lum, F.M. Torti. 1986. Possible risk of invasive pulmonary aspergillosis with marijuana use during chemotherapy for small cell lung cancer. *Drug Intell Clin Pharm* 20:289-291.

Tashkin, D.P., A.H. Coulson, V.A. Clark, M. Simmons, L.B. Bourque, S. Duann, G.H. Spivey, and H. Gong. 1987. Respiratory symptoms and lung function in habitual, heavy smokers of marijuana alone, smokers of marijuana and tobacco, smokers of tobacco alone, and nonsmokers. *Am Rev Respir Dis* 135:209-216.

Tashkin, D.P., F. Gliederer, J. Rose, P. Chang, K.K. Hui, J.L. Yu, and T-C. Wu. 1991. Effects of varying marijuana smoking profile on deposition of tar and absorption of CO and delta-9-THC. *Pharmacol Biochem Behav* 40:651-656.

Tashkin, D.P., M.S. Simmons, D. Sherrill, A.H. Coulson. 1997. Heavy habitual marijuana smoking does not cause an accelerated decline in FEV_1 with age: A longitudinal study. *Am J Respir Crit Care Med* 155:141-148.

Tashkin, D.P. 2001. Airway effects of marijuana, cocaine, and other inhaled illicit agents. *Curr Opin Pulmon Med* 7:43-61.

Taylor, D.R., R. Poulton, T.E. Moffitt, P. Ramankutty, and M.R. Sears. 2000. The respiratory effects of cannabis dependence in young adults. *Addiction* 95:1169-1677.

Tindall, B., C.R. Philpot, D.A. Cooper, J. Gold, B. Donovan, R. Penny, and T. Barnes. 1988. The Sydney AIDS project: Development of acquired immunodeficiency syndrome in a group of HIV seropositive homosexual men. *Aust NZ J Med* 18:8-15.

Ungerleider, J.T., T. Andrysiak, D.P. Tashkin, and R.P. Gale. 1982. Contamination of marihuana cigarettes with pathogenic bacteria–possible source of infection in cancer patients. *Canc Treat Rep* 66:589-591.

Wu, T-C, D.P. Tashkin, B. Djahed, and J.E. Rose. 1988. Pulmonary hazards of smoking marijuana as compared with tobacco. *N Engl J Med* 318:347-351.

Cannabis and Cannabis Extracts: Greater Than the Sum of Their Parts?

John M. McPartland

Ethan B. Russo

SUMMARY. A central tenet underlying the use of botanical remedies is that herbs contain many active ingredients. Primary active ingredients may be enhanced by secondary compounds, which act in beneficial synergy. Other herbal constituents may mitigate the side effects of dominant active ingredients. We reviewed the literature concerning medical cannabis and its primary active ingredient, Δ^9-tetrahydrocannabinol (THC). Good evidence shows that secondary compounds in cannabis may enhance the beneficial effects of THC. Other cannabinoid and non-cannabinoid compounds in herbal cannabis or its extracts may reduce THC-induced anxiety, cholinergic deficits, and immunosuppression. Cannabis terpenoids and flavonoids may also increase cerebral blood flow, enhance cortical activity, kill respiratory pathogens, and provide anti-inflammatory activity. *[Article copies available for a fee from The Haworth Document Delivery Service: 1-800-342-9678. E-mail address: <getinfo@haworthpressinc.com> Website: <http://www.HaworthPress.com> © 2001 by The Haworth Press, Inc. All rights reserved.]*

John M. McPartland, DO, MS, is affiliated with GW Pharmaceuticals, Ltd., Porton Down Science Park, Salisbury, Wiltshire, SP4 0JQ, UK.

Ethan B. Russo, MD, is affiliated with Montana Neurobehavioral Specialists, 900 North Orange Street, Missoula, MT 59802 USA.

Address correspondence to: John M. McPartland, DO, Faculty of Health & Environmental Science, UNITEC, Private Bag 92025, Auckland, New Zealand (E-mail: jmcpartland @unitec.ac.nz).

The authors thank David Pate and Vincenzo Di Marzo for pre-submission reviews.

[Haworth co-indexing entry note]: "Cannabis and Cannabis Extracts: Greater Than the Sum of Their Parts?" McPartland, John M., and Ethan B. Russo. Co-published simultaneously in *Journal of Cannabis Therapeutics* (The Haworth Integrative Healing Press, an imprint of The Haworth Press, Inc.) Vol. 1, No. 3/4, 2001, pp. 103-132; and: *Cannabis Therapeutics in HIV/AIDS* (ed: Ethan Russo) The Haworth Integrative Healing Press, an imprint of The Haworth Press, Inc., 2001, pp. 103-132. Single or multiple copies of this article are available for a fee from The Haworth Document Delivery Service [1-800-342-9678, 9:00 a.m. - 5:00 p.m. (EST). E-mail address: getinfo@haworthpressinc.com].

103

KEYWORDS. Cannabis, marijuana, THC, cannabinoids, phytocannabinoids, cannabidiol, cannabichromene, cannabibigerol, tetrahydrocannabivarin, terpenoids, essential oils, flavonoids, herbal medicine, medicinal
plants, herbal synergy

INTRODUCTION

Cannabis is an herb; it contains hundreds of pharmaceutical compounds
(Turner et al. 1980). Herbalists contend that polypharmaceutical herbs provide
two advantages over single-ingredient synthetic drugs: (1) *therapeutic effects*
of the primary active ingredients in herbs may be *synergized* by other compounds, and (2) *side effects* of the primary active ingredients may be *mitigated*
by other compounds. Thus, cannabis has been characterized as a "synergistic
shotgun," in contrast to Marinol® (Δ^9-tetrahydrocannabinol, THC), a synthetic, single-ingredient "silver bullet" (McPartland and Pruitt 1999).

Mechoulam et al. (1972) suggested that other compounds present in herbal
cannabis might influence THC activity. Carlini et al. (1974) determined that
cannabis extracts produced effects "two or four times greater than that expected from their THC content." Similarly, Fairbairn and Pickens (1981) detected the presence of unidentified "powerful synergists" in cannabis extracts
causing 330% greater activity in mice than THC alone.

Other compounds in herbal cannabis may ameliorate the side effects of
THC. Whole cannabis causes fewer psychological side effects than synthetic
THC, seen as symptoms of dysphoria, depersonalization, anxiety, panic reactions, and paranoia (Grinspoon and Bakalar 1997). This difference in side effect profiles may also be due, in part, to differences in administration: THC
taken by mouth undergoes "first pass metabolism" in the small intestine and
liver, to 11-hydroxy THC; the metabolite is more psychoactive than THC itself
(Browne and Weissman 1981). Inhaled THC undergoes little first-pass metabolism, so less 11-hydroxy THC is formed. Thus, "smoking cannabis is a satis-
factory expedient in combating fatigue, headache and exhaustion, whereas the
oral ingestion of cannabis results chiefly in a narcotic effect which may cause
serious alarm" (Walton 1938, p. 49).

Respiratory side effects from inhaling cannabis smoke may be ameliorated by
both cannabinoid and non-cannabinoid components in cannabis. For instance,
throat irritation may be diminished by anti-inflammatory agents, mutagens in
the smoke may be mitigated by antimutagens, and bacterial contaminants in
cannabis may be annulled by antibiotic compounds (McPartland and Pruitt
1997). The pharmaceutically active compounds in cannabis that enhance beneficial THC activity and reduce side effects are relatively unknown. The pur-

pose of this paper is to review the biochemistry and physiological effects of those other compounds.

MATERIALS AND METHODS

MEDLINE (1966-2000) was searched using MeSH keywords: cannabinoids, marijuana, tetrahydrocannabinol. AGRICOLA (1990-1999) was searched using the keywords cannabis, hemp, and marijuana. Phytochemical and ethnobotanical databases were searched via the Agricultural Research Service webpage <http://www.ars-grin.gov/~ngrlsb/>. All reports were scanned for supporting bibliographic citations; antecedent sources were retrieved to the fullest possible extent. Data validity was assessed by source (peer-reviewed article vs. popular press), identification methodology (analytical chemistry vs. clinical history) and the frequency of independent observations.

RESULTS AND DISCUSSION

Turner et al. (1980) listed over 420 compounds in cannabis. Sparacino et al. (1990) listed 200 additional compounds in cannabis smoke. We will highlight six cannabinoids beyond THC, a dozen-odd terpenoids, three flavonoids, and one phytosterol. Other non-cannabinoids with proven pharmacological activity include poorly characterized glycoproteins, alkaloids, and compounds that remain completely unidentified (Gill et al. 1970).

CANNABINOIDS

Mechoulam and Gaoni (1967) defined "cannabinoids" as a group of C_{21} terpenophenolic compounds uniquely produced by cannabis. The subsequent development of synthetic cannabinoids (e.g., HU-210) has blurred this definition, as has the discovery of endogenous cannabinoids (e.g., anandamide), defined as "endocannabinoids" by DiMarzo and Fontana (1995). Thus, Pate (1999) proposed the term "phytocannabinoids" to designate the C_{21} compounds produced by cannabis. Phytocannabinoids exhibit very low mammalian toxicity, and mixtures of cannabinoids are *less toxic* than pure THC (Thompson et al. 1973).

Cannabidiol (CBD) is the next-best studied phytocannabinoid after THC (Figure 1). The investigation of CBD by marijuana researchers is rather paradoxical, considering its concentrations are notably lower in drug varieties of cannabis than in fiber cultivars (Turner et al. 1980).

CBD possesses sedative properties (Carlini and Cunha, 1981), and a clinical trial showed that it reduces the anxiety and other unpleasant psychological side effects provoked by pure THC (Zuardi et al. 1982). CBD modulates the pharmacokinetics of THC by three mechanisms: (1) it has a slight affinity for cannabinoid receptors (Ki at CB1 = 4350 nM, compared to THC = 41 nM, Showalter et al. 1996), and it signals receptors as an antagonist or reverse agonist (Petitet et al. 1998), (2) CBD may modulate signal transduction by perturbing the fluidity of neuronal membranes, or by remodeling G-proteins that carry intracellular signals downstream from cannabinoid receptors, and (3) CBD is a potent inhibitor of cytochrome P450 3A11 metabolism, thus it blocks the hydroxylation of THC to its 11-hydroxy metabolite (Bornheim et al. 1995). The 11-hydroxy metabolite is four times more psychoactive than unmetabolized THC (Browne and Weissman 1981), and four times more immunosuppressive (Klein et al. 1987).

CBD provides antipsychotic benefits (Zuardi et al. 1995). It increases dopamine activity, serves as a serotonin uptake inhibitor, and enhances norepinephrine activity (Banerjee et al. 1975; Poddar and Dewey 1980). CBD protects neurons from glutamate toxicity and serves as an antioxidant, more potently than ascorbate and α-tocopherol (Hampson et al. 1998). Auspiciously, CBD does *not* decrease acetylcholine (ACh) activity in the brain (Domino 1976; Cheney et al. 1981). THC, in contrast, reduces hippocampal ACh release in rats (Carta et al. 1998), and this correlates with loss of short-term memory consolidation. In the hippocampus THC also inhibits N-methyl-D-aspartate (NMDA) receptor activity (Misner and Sullivan 1999; Shen and Thayer 1999), and NMDA synaptic transmission is crucial for memory consolidation (Shimizu et al. 2000). CBD, unlike THC, does not dampen the firing of hippocampal cells (Heyser et al. 1993) and does not disrupt learning (Brodkin and Moerschbaecher 1997).

Consroe (1998) presented an excellent review of CBD in neurological disorders. In some studies, it ameliorates symptoms of Huntington's disease, such as dystonia and dyskinesia. CBD mitigates other dystonic conditions, such as torticollis, in rat studies and uncontrolled human studies. CBD functions as an anticonvulsant in rats, on a par with phenytoin (Dilantin®, a standard antiepileptic drug).

CBD demonstrated a synergistic benefit in the reduction of intestinal motility in mice produced by THC (Anderson, Jackson, and Chesher 1974). This may be an important component of observed benefits of cannabis in inflammatory bowel diseases.

The CBD in cannabis smoke may explain why inhaling it causes less airway irritation and inflammation than inhalation of pure THC (Tashkin et al. 1977). CBD imparts analgesia (more potently than THC), it inhibits erythema (much more than THC), it blocks cyclooxygenase (COX) activity with a greater maximum inhibition than THC, and it blocks lipoxygenase (the enzyme that produces asthma-provoking leukotrienes), again more effectively than THC (Evans 1991). Mice with inflammatory collagen-induced arthritis (a mouse model for rheumatoid arthritis) were given oral CBD (5 mg/kg per day) and showed clinical improvement, and the treatment effectively blocked progression of the arthritis (Malfait et al. 2000).

CBD reportedly has little or no effect on the immune system (reviewed by Klein et al. 1998), although the mouse arthritis study by Malfait et al. (2000) showed CBD decreases the production of tumor necrosis factor (TNF) and Interferon-gamma (IFN-γ), which are two immunomodulatory cytokines described later. CBD actually kills bacteria and fungi, with greater potency than THC (Klingeren and Ham 1976; ElSohly et al. 1982; McPartland 1984). Thus, cannabis may have less microbial contamination than other herbs, an important consideration for immunocompromised individuals (McPartland and Pruitt 1997).

Cannabinol (CBN) is the degradation product of THC (Turner et al. 1980), and is found most often in aged cannabis products (Figure 1). CBN potentiates the effects of THC in man (Musty et al. 1976), yet it antagonizes the effects of THC in mice (Formukong et al. 1988). Studies reporting CBN's effects upon norepinephrine and dopamine also conflict–CBN may have negligible effects on these biogenic amines (Banerjee et al. 1975), enhance their release (Poddar and Dewey 1980), or decrease their release (Dalterio et al. 1985). CBN increases plasma concentrations of follicle-stimulating hormone, and enhances the production of testicular testosterone (Dalterio et al. 1985). CBN shares some characteristics with CBD; for example, it has anti-convulsant activity (Turner et al. 1980) and anti-inflammatory activity (Evans et al. 1991).

CBN has affinity for CB_1 receptors (Ki at CB1 = 308 nM) and signals as an agonist (Showalter et al. 1996). Further down the signal transduction cascade, it stimulates the binding of GTP-γ-S (Petitet et al. 1998), but with half the efficacy of THC; when CBN is added to THC, the effects are not significantly additive. CBN has a three-fold greater affinity for CB_2 receptors (Ki = 96 nM) (Showalter et al. 1996), thus it may affect cells of the immune system more than the central nervous system (Klein et al. 1998). CBN modulates thymocytes (Herring and Kaminski 1999) by attenuating the activity of the c-AMP response element-binding protein (CREB), nuclear factor κB (NF-κB), and interleukin-2 (IL-2). IL-2 is regulated by activator protein-1 (AP-1) transcription factor, a complex of c-Fos and c-Jun proteins (Foletta et al. 1998); CBN inhibits the expression of these proteins in splenocytes, via decreased activation of ERK MAP kinases (Faubert and Kaminski 2000).

Cannabichromene (CBC) is the fourth major cannabinoid, found predominantly in tropical *Cannabis* spp. strains (Figure 1). Until the mid-1970s, CBC was frequently misidentified as CBD, because CBC and CBD have nearly the same retention times in gas chromatography. Like CBD, CBC decreases in-flammation (Wirth et al. 1980) and provides analgesic effects (Davis and Hatoum 1983). CBC inhibits prostaglandin synthesis *in vitro*, but less potently than CBD or THC (Burstein et al. 1973). CBC exhibits strong antibacterial ac-tivity and mild antifungal activity, superior to THC and CBD in most instances (ElSohly et al. 1982). Unlike CBD, CBC has no effect on cytochrome P450 en-zymes (Kapeghian et al. 1983), nor does it function as an anticonvulsant in rats (Davis and Hatoum 1983).

The molecular affinity of CBC for cannabinoid receptors has not been mea-sured. In mice, CBC causes hypothermia, sedation, and synergizes the depres-sant effects of hexobarbital (Hatoum et al. 1981). CBC also sedates dogs and decreases muscular coordination in rats, but causes no cannabimimetic activ-ity in monkeys and people (Turner et al. 1980). In rats, the co-administration of CBC with THC potentiates THC changes in heart rate, but does not potentiate THC's hypotensive effects (O'Neil et al. 1979). Co-administration of CBC lowers the LD_{50} dose of THC in mice (Hatoum et al. 1981).

Cannabigerol (CBG) is the biosynthetic precursor of CBC, CBD, and THC, and is present only in minor amounts (Figure 1). CBG has been called "inac-tive" when compared to THC, but CBG has slight affinity for CB_1 receptors, approximately the same as CBD (Devane et al. 1988). In rat brains, CBG in-hibits the uptake of serotonin and norepinephrine, less effectively than CBD and THC, but CBG inhibits GABA uptake more effectively than CBD and THC (Banerjee et al. 1975). CBG acts as an analgesic (more potently than THC), it inhibits erythema (much more than THC), and it blocks lipoxygenase, again more effectively than THC (reviewed by Evans 1991).

CBG has antibacterial properties (Mechoulam and Gaoni 1965). Its activity against gram-positive bacteria, mycobacteria, and fungi is superior to that of THC, CBD, and CBC (ElSohly et al. 1982). CBG inhibits the growth of human oral epitheloid carcinoma cells (Baek et al. 1998).

Delta-8-THC (Δ^8-THC) is an isomer of delta-9-THC; it differs only by the location of the double bond in the cyclohexal "C" ring. The Ki of Δ^8-THC is 126 nM (Compton et al. 1993), and this loosely correlates with human studies, which show Δ^8-THC is less psychoactive than Δ^9-THC (Hollister 1974). The chemical stability of Δ^8-THC and its relative ease of synthesis compared to Δ^9-THC, have made Δ^8-THC the template for the development of two impor-tant synthetic derivatives, the extremely potent psychoactive CB_1 agonist, HU-210 (Mechoulam and Ben-Shabat 1999), and the non-psychoactive anti-emetic and neuroprotectant, HU-211 (dexanabinol) (Achiron et al. 2000; Biegon and Joseph 1995; Gallily et al. 1997). Δ^8-THC was employed clini-cally in an important study (Abrahamov and Mechoulam 1995) in which 8 children with hematological malignancies were treated with the drug over the course of 8 months at a dose of 18 mg/m^2 to treat chemotherapy-associated nausea and vomiting. Interestingly, not only was this agent uniformly effective as an antiemetic, but it was also free of psychoactive effects in this age range (2-13 years).

Tetrahydrocannabivarin (THCV) is a propyl analogue of Δ^9-THC, primarily appearing in *indica* and *afghanica* varieties of cannabis, such as hashish from Nepal (Merkus 1971), dagga from South Africa (Boucher et al. 1977), and in plants cultivated from seeds from Zambia (Pitts et al. 1992) (Figure 1). THCV is only 20-25% as psychoactive as Δ^9-THC (Hollister 1974). It has a quicker onset of action than Δ^9-THC (Gill et al. 1970), and is of briefer duration (Clarke 1998). THCV may be clinically effective in migraine treatment (Personal communication, HortaPharm, November 2000). Kubena and Barry (1972) suggested THCV synergizes the effects of THC, but did not hypothesize a mechanism. As a legal fine point, this analogue is not controlled in the Netherlands, and is not specified in the USA as a Schedule I drug, but would likely be considered illegal under the Controlled Substance Analogue Enforcement Act of 1986 (Public Law 99-570). THCV is of interest from a medical-legal standpoint in that is has been suggested as a biochemical marker of illicit cannabis use, since it is not a metabolite of Marinol® (synthetic THC) (ElSohly et al. 1999).

TERPENOIDS

The unique smell of cannabis does not arise from cannabinoids, but from over 100 terpenoid compounds (Turner et al. 1980). Terpenoids derive from repeating units of isoprene (C_5H_8), such as monoterpenoids (with C_{10} skeletons), sesquiterpenoids (C_{15}), diterpenoids (C_{20}), and triterpenoids (C_{30}). The final structure of terpenoids ranges from simple linear chains to complex polycyclic molecules, and they may include alcohol, ether, aldehyde, ketone, or ester functional groups. These compounds are easily extracted from plant material by steam distillation or vaporization. This distillate is called the *essential oil* or *volatile oil* of the plant. A range of researchers cite different yields of essential oil from different types of cannabis: Martin et al. (1961) cited yields of 0.05-0.11% essential oil from fresh, green leaves and flowers of mixed male and female plants, from feral hemp growing in Canada. Nigram et al. (1965) yielded 0.1% essential oil from fresh, whole, male plants from Kashmir. Malingré et al. (1973) yielded 0.12% essential oil from fresh leaves of "strain X" obtained from birdseed in the Netherlands. Ross and ElSohly (1996) yielded 0.29% essential oil from fresh marijuana buds, reputed to be the Afghani variety "Skunk #1." Drying the plant material led to a loss of water content and net weight, concentrating the essential oil to 0.80% in buds that had been dried at room temperature for one week (Ross and ElSohly 1966).

Field-cultivated cannabis yields about 1.3 liter of essential oil per metric ton of freshly harvested plant material (Mediavilla and Steinemann 1997). Preventing pollination increases the yield of essential oil–18 l/ha in sinsemilla crops, versus 8 l/ha in pollinated crops (Meier and Mediavilla 1998). The composition of terpenoids varies between strains of cannabis (Mediavilla and Steinemann 1997), and varies between harvest dates (Meier and Mediavilla 1998).

Many terpenoids vaporize near the same temperature as THC, which boils at 157°C (see Figures 1-2). Terpenoids are lipophilic and permeate lipid membranes. Many cross the blood-brain barrier (BBB) after inhalation (Buchbauer et al. 1993; Nasel et al. 1994).

Meschler and Howlett (1999) discussed several mechanisms by which terpenoids modulate THC activity. For instance, terpenoids may bind to cannabinoid receptors. Thujone, from *Artemisia absinthium*, has a weak affinity for CB_1 receptors (Ki at CB_1 = 130,000 nM). Terpenoids might modulate the affinity of THC for its own receptor, by sequestering THC, by perturbing annular lipids surrounding the receptor, or by increasing the fluidity of neuronal membranes. Further downstream, terpenoids may alter the signal cascade by remodeling G-proteins. Terpenoids may alter the pharmacokinetics of THC by changing the BBB; cannabis extracts are known to cause a significant increase in BBB permeability (Agrawal et al. 1989). Terpenoids may also act on other receptors and neurotransmitters. Some terpenoids act as serotonin uptake inhibitors (as does Prozac®), enhance norepinephrine activity (as do tricyclic antidepressants), increase dopamine activity (as do monoamine oxidase inhibitors and bupropion), and augment GABA (as do baclofen and the benzodiazepines). Recently, strong serotonin activity at the $5-HT_{1A}$ and $5-HT_{2a}$ receptors has been demonstrated (Russo et al. 2000; Russo 2001) that may support synergistic contributions of terpenoids on cannabis-mediated pain and mood effects. Further studies are in progress to identify the most active terpenoid components responsible, and whether synergism of the components is demonstrable.

The essential oil of cannabis is traditionally employed as an anti-inflammatory in the respiratory and digestive tracts without known contraindications at physiological dosages (Franchomme and Pénoël 1990). The essential oil of black pepper, *Piper nigrum*, has a composition of terpenes that is qualitatively quite similar to that of cannabis (Lawless 1995). It has often been claimed anecdotally, that smoked cannabis may substitute for nicotine in attempts at smoking cessation. Aside from cannabinoid influences, current evidence supports this contention based on terpene content and its activity. A recent study has shown that inhalation of black pepper essential oil vapor significantly reduced withdrawal symptoms and anxiety in tobacco smokers (Rose and Behm 1994). Interestingly, the authors posited not a central biochemical mechanism,

FIGURE 1. Phytocannabinoids

Structure*	Concentration[†] (% dry weight)	Boiling Point °C[§]	Properties
Δ-9-tetrahydrocannabinol (THC) 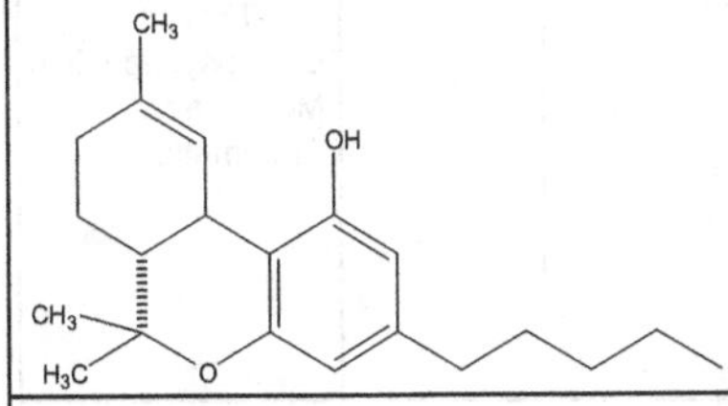 	0.1-25%	157	Euphoriant Analgesic Antiinflammatory Antioxidant Antiemetic
cannabidiol (CBD) 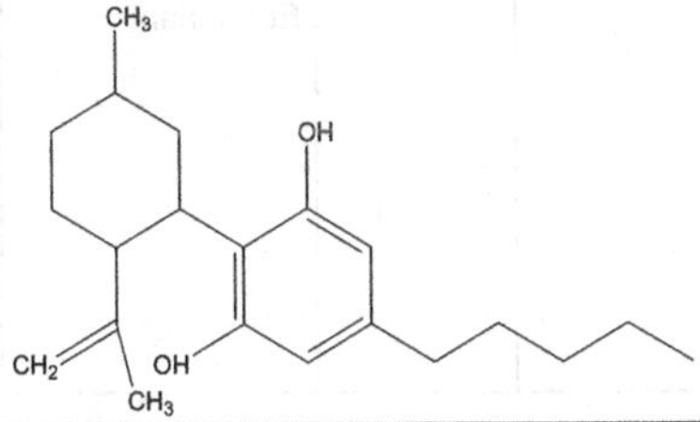 	0.1-2.89%	160-180	Anxiolytic Analgesic Antipsychotic Antiinflammatory Antioxidant Antispasmodic
cannabinol (CBN) 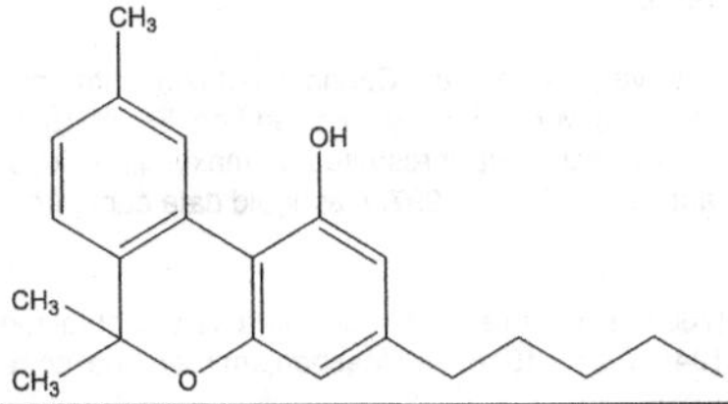 	0.0-1.6%	185	Oxidation breakdown product Sedative Antibiotic
cannabichromene (CBC) 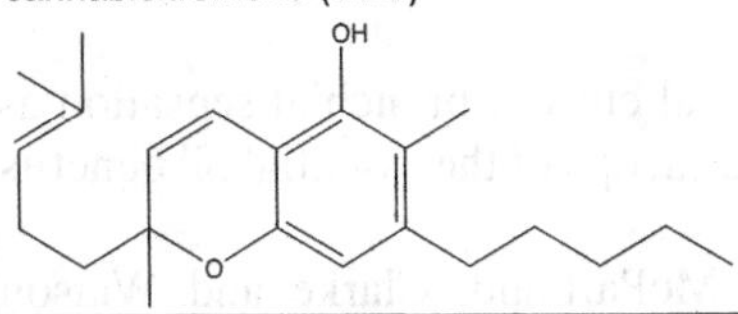 	0.0-0.65%	220	Antiinflammatory Antibiotic Antifungal
cannabigerol (CBG) 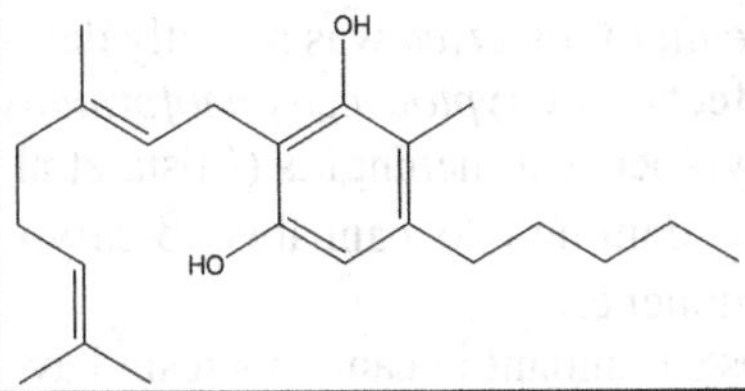 	0.03-1.15%	MP 52	Antiinflammatory Antibiotic Antifungal

FIGURE 1 (continued)

Structure*	Concentration[†] (% dry weight)	Boiling Point °C[§]	Properties
Δ-8-tetrahydrocannabinol (Δ-8-THC)	0.0-0.1%	175-178	Resembles Δ-9-THC Less psychoactive More stable Antiemetic
tetrahydrocannabivarin (THCV)	0.0-1.36%	< 220	Analgesic Euphoriant

*Structures of constituents obtained from Bissett and Wichtl 1994; British Medical Association 1997; Buckingham 1992; Iversen 2000; Tisserand and Balacs 1995; Turner et al. 1980.

[†]Concentrations of constituents (v/w or w/w) were calculated from various sources. Cannabinoid concentrations (presented as a range, including cannabinoids and cannabinoidic acids) were primarily obtained from Small, 1979; Veszki et al., 1980; Fournier et al., 1987; and Pitts et al., 1992. Terpenoid data (presented as maximum values) were calculated from Ross and El Sohly, 1996; and Mediavilla and Steinemann, 1997. Flavonoid data came from Paris et al., 1976; and Barrett et al., 1986.

[§]Boiling/melting points (MP) recorded at atmospheric pressure (760 mmHg) unless otherise noted; values obtained from various sources, primarily Buckingham, 1992; Guenther, 1948; Parry, 1918; and Mechoulam (personal communication, April 2001).

but rather a peripheral one assuming physical cues of bronchial sensation as operative in the origin of the benefit. The true scope of the essential oil benefits in this context may be quite a bit broader.

Pate (1994), McPartland (1997), and McPartland, Clarke and Watson (2000), have reviewed the pesticidal properties of cannabis attributable to its terpenoid content. The essential oil of *Eugenia dysenterica* was recently demonstrated to have significant inhibitory effects on *Cryptococcus neoformans* strains isolated from HIV patients with cryptococcal meningitis (Costa et al. 2000). Key components of that oil were common to cannabis: β-caryophyllene, α-humulene, α-terpineol, and limonene.

Additionally, monoterpenes such as those abundant in cannabis resin have been suggested to: (1) inhibit cholesterol synthesis, (2) promote hepatic en-

FIGURE 2. Terpenoid essential oil components of cannabis.

Cannabis Constituent Structure*	Concentration[†]	Boiling Point °C[§]	Properties
β-myrcene 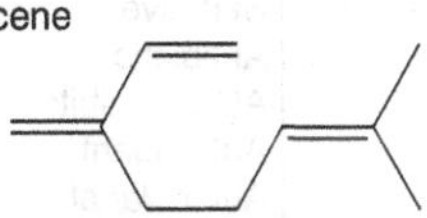	0.47%	166-168	Analgesic Antiinflammatory Antibiotic Antimutagenic
β-caryophyllene 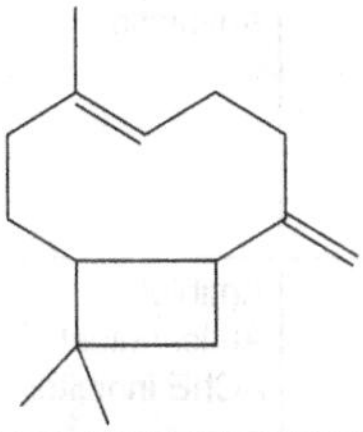	0.05%	119	Antiinflammatory Cytoprotective (gastric mucosa) Antimalarial
d-limonene 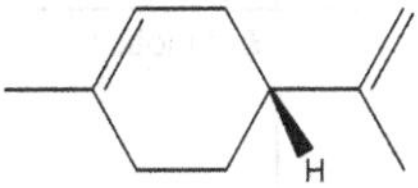	0.14%	177	Cannabinoid agonist? Immune potentiator Antidepressant Antimutagenic
linalool 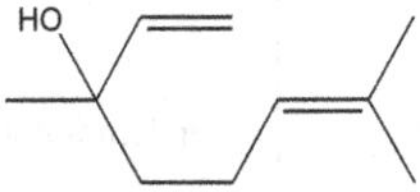	0.002%	198	Sedative Antidepressant Anxiolytic Immune potentiator
pulegone 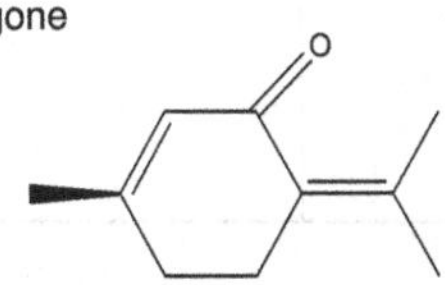	0.001%	224	Memory booster? AChE inhibitor Sedative Antipyretic
1,8-cineole (eucalyptol) 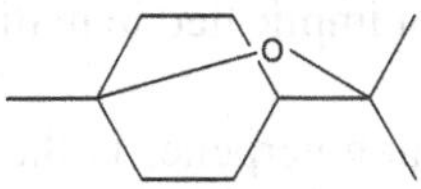	> 0.001%	176	AChE inhibitor Increases cerebral blood flow Stimulant Antibiotic Antiviral Antiinflammatory Antinociceptive
α-pinene 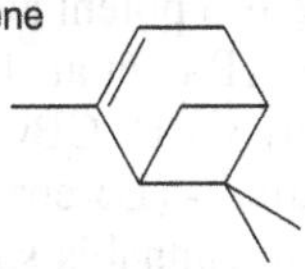	0.04%	156	Antiinflammatory Bronchodilator Stimulant Antibiotic Antineoplastic AChE inhibitor

FIGURE 2 (continued)

Cannabis Constituent Structure*	Concentration[†]	Boiling Point °C[§]	Properties
α-terpineol 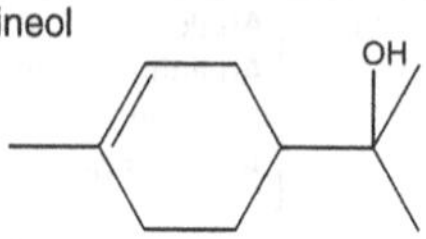	0.02%	217-218	Sedative Antibiotic AChE inhibitor Antioxidant Antimalarial
terpineol-4-ol 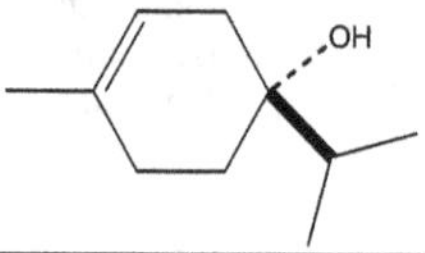	0.0004%	209	AChE inhibitor Antibiotic
p-cymene 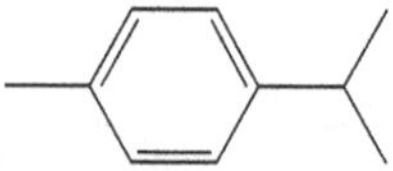	0.0004%	177	Antibiotic Anticandidal AChE inhibitor
borneol 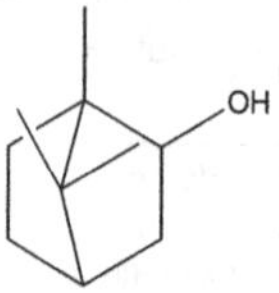	0.008%	210	Antibiotic
Δ-3-carene 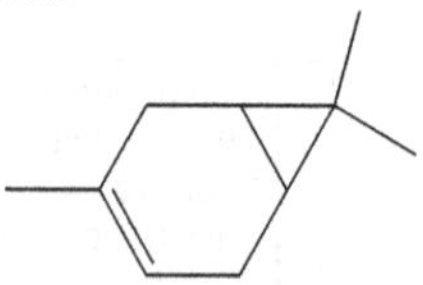	0.004%	168	Antiinflammatory

zyme activity to detoxify carcinogens, (3) stimulate apoptosis in cells with damaged DNA, and (4) inhibit protein isoprenylation implicated in malignant deterioration (Jones 1999).

Myrcene, specifically β-myrcene, a noncyclic monoterpene, is the most abundant terpenoid produced by cannabis (Ross and ElSohly 1996; Mediavilla and Steinemann 1997). It also occurs in high concentrations in hops (*Humulus lupulus*) and lemongrass (*Cymbopogon citratus*). Myrcene is a potent analgesic, acting at central sites that are antagonized by naloxone (Rao et al. 1990). Myrcene also works via a peripheral mechanism shared by CBD, CBG, and CBC–by blocking the inflammatory activity of prostaglandin E_2 (Lorenzetti et al. 1991). This activity is expressed by other terpenoids in cannabis smoke, such as carvacrol, which is more potent than THC or CBG (Burstein et al. 1975). The activity of many terpenoids may be cumulative: unfractionated cannabis essential oil exhibits greater antiinflammatory activity than its individual constituents, suggesting synergy (Evans et al. 1987).

Myrcene also synergizes the antibiotic potency of other essential oil components, against *Staphylococcus aureus, Bacillus subtilis, Pseudomonas aeruginosa,* and a specific strain of *Escherichia coli* (Onawunmi et al. 1984). Myrcene inhibits cytochrome P450 2B1, an enzyme implicated in the metabolic activation of promutagens (De Oliveira et al. 1997). Aflatoxin B_1 is a promutagen produced by *Aspergillus flavus* and *Aspergillus parasiticus,* two fungal contaminants of moldy marijuana (reviewed by McPartland and Pruitt 1997). After aflatoxin B_1 is metabolized by P450 2B1, it becomes extremely hepatocarcinogenic. Myrcene blocks this metabolism, as do other terpenoids in cannabis, including limonene, α-pinene, α-terpinene, and citronellal (De Oliveira et al. 1997).

β-Caryophyllene is the most common sesquiterpenoid in cannabis (Mediavilla and Steinemann 1997). It is the main component of copaiba balsam, from *Copaifera* spp. (Lawless 1995), which is a popular oral and topical anti-inflammatory agent in Brazil (Basile et al. 1988). The latter authors were able to demonstrate anti-inflammatory effects of the oleoresin in rats comparable to phenylbutazone, in reduction of granuloma formation. A decreased vascular permeability to injected histamine was also observed.

A gastric cytoprotective effect of β-caryophyllene was demonstrated in rats against challenge with absolute ethanol and hydrochloric acid (Tambe et al. 1996). This benefit was noted without influence on gastric acid or pepsin secretion. The authors suggested this agent as clinically safe, and potentially useful. Campbell et al. (1997) have demonstrated a moderate antimalarial effect against two strains of *Plasmodium falciparum* by an essential oil rich in β-caryophyllene and α-terpineol.

Limonene is a monocyclic monoterpenoid and a major constituent of citrus rinds (Tisserand and Balacs 1995). It finds extensive use as a solvent and in the perfumery and flavor industries. Because of limonene's widespread occurrence and application, its biological activity is well known. Limonene is highly absorbed by inhalation and quickly appears in the bloodstream (Falk-Flilipsson et al. 1993). According to Ross and ElSohly (1996), limonene is the second most common terpenoid in an unidentified cultivar of cannabis.

Limonene may have a low-affinity interaction with cannabinoid receptors (Meschler and Howlett 1999). Studies of long-term inhalation of lemon fragrance (predominately limonene) have demonstrated inhibition of thymic involution in stress-induced immunosuppression in mice (Ortiz de Urbina et al. 1989).

Limonene was the primary component of the essential oil mixture employed by Komori et al. (1995), in their clinical study of immune function and depressive states in humans. The key result of this experiment was the ability to markedly reduce the dosage of, or even eliminate the need for, synthetic antidepressant drugs.

As mentioned in the myrcene section, limonene protects against aflatoxin B_1-induced cancer by inhibiting the hepatic metabolism of the promutagen to its active form. Limonene also blocks this process at two earlier steps by inhibiting the growth of *Aspergillus* fungi and inhibiting their production of aflatoxins (Greene-McDowelle et al. 1999). Limonene and other terpenoids suppress the growth of many species of fungi and bacteria, demonstrated in hundreds of published studies (reviewed by McPartland 1997).

Limonene blocks the carcinogenesis induced by benz[α]anthracene (Crowell 1999), a component of the "tar" generated by the combustion of herbal cannabis. Thus, this terpenoid may reduce the harm caused by inhaling cannabis smoke. Limonene blocks carcinogenesis by multiple mechanisms. It detoxifies carcinogens by inducing Phase II carcinogen-metabolizing enzymes (Crowell 1999). It selectively inhibits the isoprenylation of Ras proteins, thus blocking the action of mutant *ras* oncogenes (Hardcastle et al. 1999). It induces redifferentiation of cancer cells (by enhancing expression of transforming growth factor β1 and growth factor II receptors), and it induces apoptosis of cancer cells (Crowell 1999). Orally administered limonene is currently undergoing Phase II clinical trials in the treatment of breast cancer (Vigushin et al. 1998); it also protects against lung, liver, colon, pancreas, and skin cancers (Vigushin et al. 1998; Crowell 1999; Setzer et al. 1999).

Linalool is a noncyclic monoterpenoid, commonly extracted from lavender (*Lavandula* spp.), rose (*Rosa* spp.), and neroli oil (from *Citrus aurantium*). It usually constitutes 5% or less of cannabis essential oil (Ross and ElSohly 1996). Linalool nevertheless exhibits strong biological activity. Buchbauer et al. (1993) assayed the sedative effects of over 40 terpenoids upon *inhalation* by mice; linalool was the most powerful, reducing mouse motility 73% after 1 hour of inhalation. The study demonstrated that other terpenoids found in cannabis, such as citronellol and α-terpineol, are also deeply sedating upon inhalation, even in low concentrations. Furthermore, combinations of these terpenoids (e.g., neroli oil) are synergistic in their sedative effects. These terpenoids may mitigate the anxiety provoked by pure THC. Inhalation of such terpenoids also provides antidepressant effects (Komori et al. 1995).

Reducing anxiety and depression will improve immune function via the neuroendocrine system, by damping down the hypothalamic-pituitary-adrenal (HPA) axis. Hence, inhalation of terpenoids reduces the secretion of HPA stress hormones (e.g., corticosterone), and normalizes CD4-CD8 ratios (Komori et al. 1995). By a similar mechanism, terpenoids in *Ginkgo biloba* inhibit corticosterone secretion by attenuating corticotropin-releasing factor (CRF) expression (Marcihac et al. 1998). CRF not only induces corticosterone secretion via the HPA axis, it is also associated with anxiety. Rodríguez de Fonseca et al. (1996) showed that the psychoactive cannabinoid HU-210 caused a release of CRF. Thus, the terpenoids act synergistically with non-psychoactive CBD, which may decrease CRF by inhibiting IFN-γ (Malfait et al. 2000).

Pulegone, a monocyclic monoterpenoid, is a minor constituent of cannabis (Turner et al. 1980). Higher concentrations of pulegone are found in rosemary (*Rosmarinus officinalis*), "the herb of remembrance." Pulegone may alleviate a major side effect of THC–loss of short-term memory consolidation. THC causes acetylcholine (ACh) deficits in the hippocampus. Hippocampal ACh deficits are also seen in people with Alzheimer's disease. Alzheimer's patients can be treated with tacrine (Cognex®), a drug that increases ACh activity by inhibiting acetylcholinesterase (AChE). Indeed, tacrine has blocked THC-induced memory loss behavior in rats. Pulegone exhibits the same activity as tacrine, that of AChE inhibition (Miyazawa et al. 1997). Other terpenoids in cannabis also provide AChE inhibition, including limonene, limonene oxide, α-terpinene, γ-terpinene, terpinen-4-ol, carvacrol, l-and d-carvone, 1,8-cineole, *p*-cymene, fenchone, and pulegone-1,2-epoxide (Perry et al. 1996; McPartland and Pruitt 1999). The beneficial effects of AChE inhibitors, however, are decreased in individuals carrying the E4 subtype of the apolipoprotein E gene, ApoE E4 (Poirier et al. 1995). Pulegone has also demonstrated significant sedative and antipyretic properties in a study in rats (Ortiz de Urbina et al. 1989).

1,8-Cineole, a bicyclic monoterpenoid, is a minor constituent of cannabis and the major aromatic found in *Eucalyptus* species. Studies show the inhalation of 1,8-cineole increases cerebral blood flow and enhances cortical activity (Nasel et al. 1994). Brain function is enhanced by administering terpenoids that improve cerebral blood flow, much as the ginkgolides in *Ginkgo biloba* (Russo 2000). Similarly, cerebral blood flow increases after inhaling cannabis smoke, and this increase is *not* related to plasma levels of THC (Mathew and Wilson 1993).

A stimulatory effect on rat locomotion was demonstrated employing a 1,8-cineole-rich essential oil of rosemary with a terpene profile similar to that of cannabis (Kovar et al. 1987). Blood levels correlated with the degree of stimulation observed. Antinociceptive and anti-inflammatory effects of 1,8-cineole were demonstrated at high doses in rats, using carrageenan rat paw and cotton pellet-induced granuloma models (Santos and Rao 2000). An analgesic effect of an essential oil was demonstrated in another animal study, and correlated with the 1,8-cineole concentration (Aydin et al. 1999).

1,8-Cineole demonstrated antibacterial activity against *Bacillus subtilis*, and antifungal properties against *Trichophyton mentagrophytes*, *Cryptococcus neoformans*, and *Candida albicans* (Hammerschmidt et al. 1993). In subsequent assays, this essential oil component was cidal against *Candida albicans* and *Escherichia coli*, and bacteriostatic against *Staphylococcus aureus* (Carson and Riley 1995). In a rat study, 1,8-cineole prevented the sexual transmission of *Herpes simplex* virus type 2 (HSV-2). HSV-2 is a frequently comorbid condition with HIV, and its prevention has been suggested as one method of lowering HIV transmission risks (Gwanzura et al. 1998).

Perry et al. (2000) demonstrated that 1,8-cineole was an inhibitor of human erythrocyte acetylcholinesterase, but that an essential oil of *Salvia lavandulaefolia* containing 1,8-cineole and other terpenoids produced a synergistic inhibition of acetylcholinesterase that suggested utility in the clinical treatment of Alzheimer's disease. A similar mechanism may operate in cannabis essential oil with the same components.

α-Pinene, a bicyclic monoterpenoid, was effective in prevention of acute inflammation in a carrageenan-induced plantar edema model (Gil et al. 1989). A pharmacokinetics study of inhaled α-pinene in humans demonstrated 60% uptake, and a relative bronchodilation effect (Falk et al. 1990). After 1 hour of inhalation, α-pinene produced a 13.8% increase in mouse motility measures (Buchbauer et al. 1993). α-Pinene has inhibited acetylcholinesterase in a variety of assays (Perry et al. 1996; McPartland and Pruitt 1999), suggesting utility in the clinical treatment of Alzheimer's disease. The antibiotic properties of α-pinene, α-terpineol, and terpinen-4-ol have been demonstrated against *Staphylococcus aureus, S. epidermidis* and *Propionibacterium acnes* (Raman et al. 1995). α-Pinene and its isomer β-pinene were both cytotoxic *in vitro* against Hep-G2 (human hepatocellular carcinoma) and Sk-Mel-28 (human melanoma) tumor cell lines (Setzer et al. 1999).

α-Terpineol, terpinen-4-ol, and 4-terpineol are three closely related monoterpenoids. Inhalation of α-terpineol reduced mouse motility 45% (Buchbauer et al. 1993). Burits and Bucar (2000) demonstrated that 4-terpineol exhibits "respectable" radical scavenging and antioxidant properties. Terpinen-4-ol, α-terpineol, and α-pinene demonstrated dose-dependent antibiotic properties against *Staphylococcus aureus, S. epidermidis* and *Propionibacterium acnes* (Raman et al. 1995). Similar studies have demonstrated antimicrobial activity against a wide range of pathogenic organisms, excluding *Pseudomonas* (Carson and Riley 1995). Campbell et al. (1997) have demonstrated a moderate antimalarial effect against two strains of *Plasmodium falciparum* by an essential oil with major α-terpineol and α-caryophyllene components.

Cymene, or *p*-cymene, a monoterpenoid, is active against *Bacterioides fragilis, Candida albicans*, and *Clostridium perfringens* (Carson and Riley 1995).

Borneol, a bicyclic monoterpenoid, was tested in walnut oil as an external treatment for purulent otitis media (Liu 1990), where it proved to be 98% effective (P < 0.001), to a greater degree than neomycin, and without toxicity.

Δ^3-Carene, a bicyclic monoterpenoid, was effective in prevention of acute inflammation in a carrageenan-induced plantar edema model (Gil et al. 1989).

FLAVONOIDS

Flavonoids are aromatic, polycyclic phenols. Cannabis produces about 20 of these compounds, as free flavonoids and conjugated glycosides (Turner et al. 1980). Paris et al. (1976) estimated that cannabis leaves consist of 1% flavonoids. Some flavonoids are volatile, lipophilic, permeate membranes, and apparently retain pharmacological activity in cannabis smoke (Sauer et al. 1983). Flavonoids may modulate the pharmacokinetics of THC, via a mechanism shared by CBD, the inhibition of P450 3A11 and P450 3A4 enzymes. Naringenin, a flavonoid in grapefruit juice, also inhibits these enzymes, thus blocking the metabolism of cyclosporine, caffeine, benzodiazepines, and calcium antagonists (Fuhr 1998). Two related enzymes, P450 3A4 and P450 1A1, metabolize environmental toxins from procarcinogens to their activated forms. Thus, P450-suppressing compounds serve as chemoprotective agents, shielding healthy cells from the activation of benzo[α]pyrene and aflatoxin B_1 (Offord et al. 1997), which are two procarcinogens potentially found in cannabis smoke (McPartland and Pruitt 1997).

Apigenin is a flavone found in nearly all vascular plants (Figure 3). It exerts a wide range of biological effects, including many properties shared by terpenoids and cannabinoids. Apigenin is the primary anxiolytic agent found in chamomile, *Matricaria recutita*, (reviewed in Russo 2000). It selectively binds with high affinity to central benzodiazepine receptors, which are located in α- and β-subunits of GABA$_A$ receptors (Salgueiro et al. 1997); this anxiolytic activity is not associated with the unwanted side effects caused by synthetic benzodiazepines, such as muscular relaxation, amnesia, and sedation.

Apigenin inhibits the production of tumor necrosis factor-alpha (TNF-α), a cytokine primarily expressed by monocytes and macrophages (Gerritsen et al. 1995). TNF-α induces and maintains inflammation, a pathological condition in rheumatoid arthritis and multiple sclerosis. THC decreases TNF-α, probably by a nonreceptor-mediated mechanism (Burnette-Curley and Cabral 1995), although one study suggested THC might induce TNF-α (Shivers et al. 1994). Either way, apigenin provides beneficial suppression of TNF-α, whether in concert with THC or counteracting THC.

FIGURE 3. Flavonoid and phytosterol components of cannabis.

Cannabis Constituent Structure*	Concentration[†]	Boiling Point °C[§]	Properties
apigenin 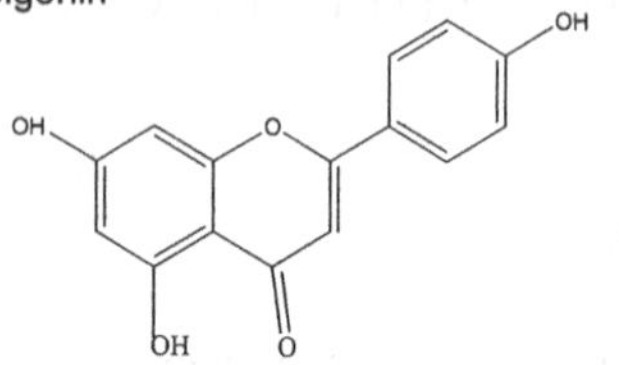	> 0.1%	178	Anxiolytic Antiinflammatory Estrogenic
quercetin 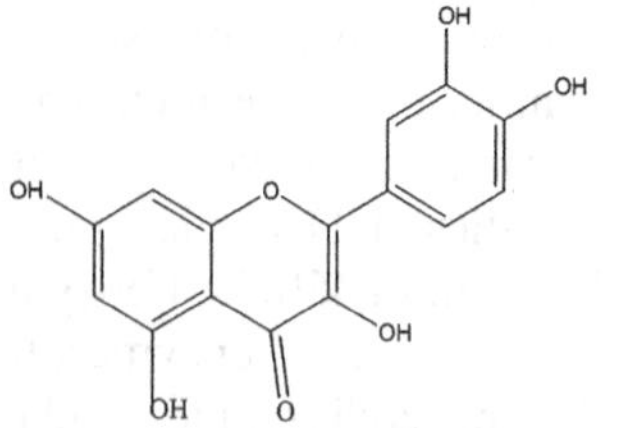	> 0.1%	250	Antioxidant Antimutagenic Antiviral Antineoplastic
cannflavin A 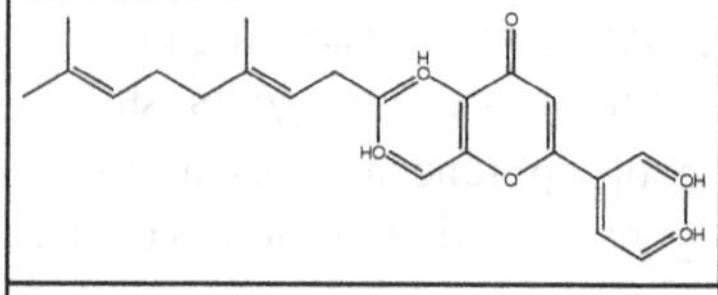	0.02%	182	COX inhibitor LO inhibitor
β-sitosterol 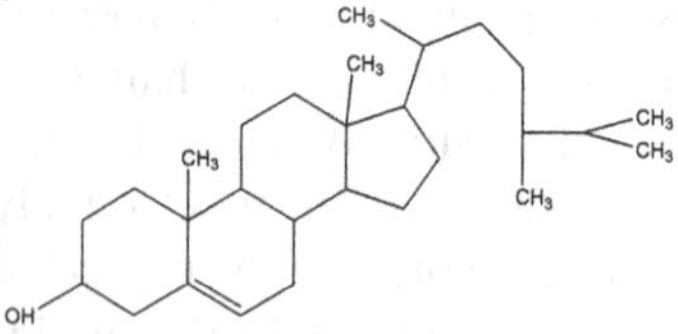	?	134	Antiinflammatory 5-α-reductase inhibitor

Apigenin and other flavonoids interact with estrogen receptors, and appear to be the primary estrogenic agents in cannabis smoke (Sauer et al. 1983). Although apigenin has a high affinity for estrogen receptors (especially β-estrogen receptors), it has low estrogenic activity; apigenin actually inhibits estradiol-induced proliferation of breast cancer cells (Wang and Kurzer 1998).

Quercetin is a flavonol found in nearly all vascular plants, including cannabis (Turner et al. 1980). Quercetin is a potent antioxidant; by some measures more potent than ascorbic acid, α-tocopherol, and BHT (Gadow et al. 1997). Combinations of quercetin and other antioxidants work synergistically (Hudson and Mahgoub 1981). The antioxidant potential of quercetin and other flavonoids should be tested against CBD, another potent antioxidant (Hampson et al. 1998). Perhaps flavonoids can induce chemical reduction of CBD, effectively recycling CBD as an antioxidant. Flavonoids block free radical formation at several steps: by scavenging superoxide anions (in both enzymatic and non-enzymatic systems), by quenching intermediate peroxyl and alkoxyl radicals, and by chelating iron ions, which catalyze many Fenton reactions leading to free radical formation (Musonda and Chipman 1998).

Free radicals activate NF-κB, a transcription factor protein that induces the expression of oncogenes, inflammation, and apoptosis. Quercetin arrests the formation of NF-κB, by blocking the PKC-induced phosphorylation of an inhibitory subunit of NF-κB called IκB (Musonda and Chipman 1998), consequently quercetin hinders carcinogenesis and inflammatory diseases. NF-κB also plays a role in the activation of HIV-1 (Greenspan 1993), so quercetin may hinder the replication of that virus. In a similar fashion, silymarin (a flavonoid produced by milk thistle, *Silybum marianum*) impedes NF-κB-induced replication of the hepatitis C virus, and thus inhibits hepatic carcinoma (McPartland 1996). These flavonoids may synergize with CBN, which also downregulates NF-κB (Herring and Kaminski 1999), thereby counteracting the effects of THC, which may increase NF-κB activity (Daaka et al. 1997).

Cannflavin A is one of a pair of prenylated flavones apparently unique to cannabis (Barrett et al. 1986). The yield of cannflavin A is 0.02% of dry herb. This compound is a potent inhibitor of prostaglandin E_2 in human rheumatoid synovial cells, with an IC_{50} of 31 ng/ml, about 30 times more potent than aspirin in that system (Barrett et al. 1986). Cannflavin A inhibits cyclooxygenase (COX) enzymes and lipoxygenase (LO) enzymes more potently than THC (Evans et al. 1987). However, these assays were done with alcohol-extracted cannflavin; we question whether cannflavin is sufficiently volatile. Other phenols related to flavonoids are volatile and apparently retain pharmacological activity in cannabis smoke, such as eugenol and *p*-vinylphenol (Burstein et al. 1976).

β-Sitosterol was demonstrated in significant concentrations in the red oil extract of cannabis (Fenselau and Hermann 1972). In animal assays, this phytosterol reduced acute inflammation 65% and chronic edema 40.6% (Gomez et al. 1999). This agent has been the subject of most interest as the active ingredient of *Serenoa repens*, the saw palmetto, and *Urtica dioica*, the nettle, wherein β-sitosterol acts as a 5-α-reductase inhibitor. In numerous trials (Wilt et al. 1998; McPartland and Pruitt 2000), standardized extracts of saw palmetto have proven equivalent or superior to finasteride in treatment of benign prostatic hyperplasia.

CONCLUSIONS

Does the body absorb non-cannabinoids in physiologically relevant concentrations? In the absence of experimental data, we can estimate, using limonene as an example of AChE inhibition. According to Ross and ElSohly (1996), fresh, female flowering tops consist of 0.29% essential oil. Air drying of female flowering tops decreases their moisture content (MC) from approximately 85% MC to 15% MC, with a concomitant loss in water weight (McPartland and Pruitt 1997). Although some essential oil is volatilized and lost in the drying process, the remaining terpenoids become concentrated. The concentration of essential oil in air-dried cannabis is 0.8%, and limonene consists of 17.2% of the essential oil (Ross and ElSohly 1996). Thus, air-dried cannabis consists of 0.14% limonene; therefore a 500 mg cannabis cigarette (which is half the size of a standard tobacco cigarette) would contain 0.7 mg limonene. If we assume the systemic bioavailability of limonene from smoking cannabis is 18%, the same as THC (Ohlsson et al. 1980), then 0.13 mg would be absorbed. Distributing this dose evenly in the total body water of a 70 kg man, without metabolism or sequestration, would produce a maximum tissue concentration of 1.3 μM. This concentration is an order of magnitude below the IC_{50} concentration of limonene's inhibition of AChE (Miyazawa et al. 1997). Hence, limonene *must* synergize with other AChE inhibitors in order to be effective.

Vaporizer technology may improve the bioavailability of limonene and other compounds, which volatilize around the same temperature as THC (see Figures 1-3). Vaporizers are smoking apparati that heat cannabis to 185°C (365°F), which vaporizes THC but is below the ignition point of combustible plant material. Vaporized cannabis emits a thin gray vapor, whereas combusted cannabis produces a thick smoke. Thus, vaporizers deliver a better cannabinoid-to-tar ratio than cigarettes or water pipes (Gieringer 1996). In a recent study, traces of THC were vaporized at temperatures as low as 140°C (284°F) and the majority of THC vaporized by 185°C (365°F); benzene and other carcinogenic vapors did not appear until 200°C (392°F), and cannabis combustion occurred around 230°C (446°F) (Gieringer 2001).

Concerning bioavailability, it should be mentioned that cannabis compounds need not be absorbed systemically through the lungs to produce CNS activity. Inhaled compounds may reach receptors in the olfactory bulb, sending mood-altering messages via olfactory nerves directly to the limbic region and hippocampus. This route may be responsible for some sedative effects of terpenoids upon inhalation (Buchbauer et al. 1993).

The paucity of research concerning non-THC synergists in cannabis is periodically criticized (Mechoulam et al. 1972; McPartland and Pruitt 1999; Russo 2000). We have highlighted several cannabinoids, terpenoids, and flavonoids that deserve further attention regarding their contributions to the effects of clinical cannabis. Most of the data we present here is based on *in vitro* experiments or animal studies. Clearly the next step should involve human clinical trials of each constituent, alone, or in combination with THC, or combined with a cocktail of cannabis compounds.

REFERENCES

Abrahamov, A., and R. Mechoulam. 1995. An efficient new cannabinoid antiemetic in pediatric oncology. *Life Sci* 56(23-24):2097-102.

Achiron, A., S. Miron, V. Lavie, R. Margalit, and A. Biegon. 2000. Dexanabinol (HU-211) effect on experimental autoimmune encephalomyelitis: implications for the treatment of acute relapses of multiple sclerosis. *J Neuroimmunol* 102(1):26-31.

Agrawal, A.K., P. Kumar, A. Gulati, and P.K. Seth. 1989. Cannabis-induced neurotoxicity in mice: effects on cholinergic (muscarinic) receptors and blood brain barrier permeability. *Res Commun Subst Abuse* 10:155-68.

Anderson, P.F., D.M. Jackson, and G.B. Chesher. 1974. Interaction of delta-9-tetrahydrocannabinol and cannabidiol on intestinal motility in mice. *J Pharm Pharmacol* 26(2):136-7.

Aydin, S., T. Demir, Y. Ozturk, and K.H. Baser. 1999. Analgesic activity of *Nepeta italica* L. *Phytother Res* 13(1):20-3.

Baek, S.H., Y.O. Kim, J.S. Kwag, K.E. Choi, W.Y. Jung, and D.S. Han. 1998. Boron trifluoride etherate on silica-A modified Lewis acid reagent (VII). Antitumor activity of cannabigerol against human oral epitheloid carcinoma cells. *Arch Pharmacol Res* 21:353-6.

Banerjee, S.P., S.H. Snyder, R. Mechoulam. 1975. Cannabinoids: influence on neurotransmitter uptake in rat brain synaptosomes. *J Pharmacol Exper Therap* 194:74-81.

Barrett, M.L., A.M. Scutt, and F.J. Evans. 1986. Cannflavin A and B, prenylated flavones from *Cannabis sativa* L. *Experientia* 42:452-3.

Basile, A.C., J.A. Sertie, P.C. Freitas, and A.C. Zanini. 1988. Anti-inflammatory activity of oleoresin from Brazilian *Copaifera*. *J Ethnopharmacol* 22(1):101-9.

Biegon, A., and A.B. Joseph. 1995. Development of HU-211 as a neuroprotectant for ischemic brain damage. *Neurol Res* 17(4):275-80.

Bisset, N.G. and M. Wichtl. 1994. *Herbal drugs and phytopharmaceuticals: A handbook for practice on a scientific basis*. Stuttgart, Boca Raton: Medpharm Scientific Publishers, CRC Press.

Bornheim, L.M., K.Y. Kim, J. Li, B.Y. Perotti, and L.Z. Benet. 1995. Effect of cannabidiol pretreatment on the kinetics of tetrahydrocannabinol metabolites in mouse brain. *Drug Metab Dispos* 23:825-31.

Boucher, F., M. Paris, and L. Cosson. 1977. Mise en évidence de deux type chimques chez le *Cannabis sativa* originaire d'Afrique du Sud. *Phytochem* 16:1445-8.

British Medical Association. 1997. *Therapeutic uses of cannabis*. Amsterdam: Harwood Academic Publishers.

Brodkin, J., and J.M. Moerschbaecher. 1997. SR141716A antagonizes the disruptive effects of cannabinoid ligaands on learning in rats. *J Pharmacol Exper Therap* 282:1526-32.

Browne, R.G., and A. Weissman. 1981. Discriminative stimulus properties of delta 9-tetrahydrocannabinol: mechanistic studies. *J Clin Pharmacol* 21(8-9 Suppl): 227S-34S.

Buchbauer, G., L. Jirovetz, W. Jager, C. Plank, and H. Dietrich. 1993. Fragrance compounds and essential oils with sedative effects upon inhalation. *J Pharm Sci* 82(6):660-4.

Buckingham, J., editor. 1992. *Dictionary of natural products*. London: Chapman & Hall.

Burits, M., and F. Bucar. 2000. Antioxidant activity of *Nigella sativa* essential oil. *Phytoth Res* 14(5):323-8.

Burnette-Curley, D., and G.A. Cabral. 1995. Differential inhibition of RAW264.7 macrophage tumoricidal activity by Δ^9-tetrahydrocannabinol. *Proc Soc Exp Biol Med* 210:64-76.

Burstein, S., C. Varanelli, and L.T. Slade. 1975. Prostaglandins and *Cannabis*–III. Inhibition of biosynthesis by essential oil components of marihuana. *Biochemical Pharmacology* 24:1053-4.

Burstein, S., E. Levin, and C. Varanelli. 1973. Prostaglandins and *Cannabis*–II. Inhibition of biosynthesis by the naturally occurring cannabinoids. *Biochem Pharmacol* 22:2905-10.

Burstein, S., P. Taylor, F.S. El-Feraly, C. Turner. 1976. Prostaglandins and *Cannabis*–V. Identification of p-vinylphenol as a potent inhibitor of prostaglandin synthesis. *Biochem Pharmacol* 25:2003-4.

Campbell, W.E., D.W. Gammon, P. Smith, M. Abrahams, and T.D. Purves. 1997. Composition and antimalarial activity *in vitro* of the essential oil of *Tetradenia riparia*. *Planta Med* 63(3):270-2.

Carlini, E.A., and J.M. Cunha. 1981. Hypnotic and antiepileptic effects of cannabidiol. *J Clin Pharmacol* 21:417S-27S.

Carlini, E.A., I.G. Karniol, P.F. Renault, and C.R. Schuster. 1974. Effects of marihuana in laboratory animals and man. *Brit J Pharmacol* 50:299-309.

Carson, C.F., and T.V. Riley. 1995. Antimicrobial activity of the major components of the essential oil of *Melaleuca alternifolia*. *J Appl Bacter* 78(3):264-9.

Carta, G., F. Nava, and G.L. Gessa. 1998. Inhibition of hippocampal acetylcholine release after acute and repeated Δ^9-tetrahydrocannabinol in rats. *Brain Res* 809:1-4.

Cheney, D.L., A.V. Revuelta, and E. Costa. Marijuana and cholinergic dynamics. In G. Pepeu and H. Ladinsky, eds., 1981. *Cholinergic mechanisms: Phylogenetic aspects, central and peripheral synapses, and clinical significance*. New York: Plenum Press.

Clarke, R.C. 1998. *Hashish!* Los Angeles, CA: Red Eye Press.

Compton, D.R., K.C. Rice, B.R. DeCosta, R.K. Razdan, L.S. Melvin, M.R. Johnson, and B.R. Martin. 1993. Cannabinoid structure-activity relationships: correlation of receptor binding and *in vivo* activities. *J Pharmacol Exp Therap* 265:218-26.

Consroe, P. 1998. Brain cannabinoid systems as targets for the therapy of neurological disorders. *Neurobiol Dis* 5:534-51.

Costa, T.R., O.F. Fernandes, S.C. Santos, C.M. Oliveira, L.M. Liao, P.H. Ferri, J.R. Paula, H.D. Ferreira, B.H. Sales, and M.R. Silva. 2000. Antifungal activity of volatile constituents of *Eugenia dysenterica* leaf oil. *J Ethnopharmacol* 72(1-2): 111-7.

Crowell, P.L. 1999. Prevention and therapy of cancer by dietary monoterpenes. *J Nutr* 1999; 129:775S-8S.

Daaka, Y., W. Zhu, H. Friedman, and T.W. Klein. 1997. Induction of interleukin-2 receptor α gene by Δ^9-tetrahydrocannabinol is mediated by nuclear factor κB and CB1 cannabinoid receptor. *DNA Cell Biol* 16:301-9.

Dalterio, S., D. Mayfield, A. Bartke, W. Morgan. 1985. Effects of psychoactive and non-psychoactive cannabinoids on neuroendocrine and testicular responsiveness in mice. *Life Sci* 36:1299-306.

Davis, W.M., and N.S. Hatoum. 1993. Neurobehavioral actions of cannabichromene and interactions with Δ^9-tetrahydrocannabinol. *Gen Pharmacol* 14(2):247-52.

De Oliverira, A.C., L.F. Ribeiro-Pinto, J.R. Paumgartten. 1997. *In vitro* inhibition of CYP2B1 monooxygenase by beta-myrcene and other monoterpenoid compounds. *Toxicol Lett* 92:39-46.

Devane, W.A., F.A. Dysarz, M.R. Johnson, L.S. Melvin, A.C. Howlett. 1998. Determination and characterization of a cannabinoid receptor in rat brain. *Molecular Pharmacol* 34:605-13.

Di Marzo, V. and A. Fontana. 1995. Anandamide, an endogenous cannabinomimetic eicosanoid: "killing two birds with one stone." *Prostagland Leukotr Essent Fatty Acids* 53:1-11.

Domino, E.F. 1976. Effect of Δ^9-terahydrocannabinol and cannabinol on rat brain acetylcholine. In Nahas G.G., Panton W.D.M., Idanpaan-Heikkila J.E., eds. *Marijuana: chemistry, biochemistry, and cellular effects.* New York: Springer-Verlag: pp. 407-13.

ElSohly, H.N., C.E. Turner, A.M. Clark, and M.A. ElSohly. 1982. Synthesis and antimicrobial activities of certain cannabichromene and cannabigerol related compounds. *J Pharmaceut Sci* 71:1319-23.

ElSohly, M.A., S. Feng, T.P. Murphy, S.A. Ross, A. Nimrod, Z. Mehmedic, and N. Fortner. 1999. Delta-9-tetrahydrocannabivarin (delta-9-THCV) as a marker for the ingestion of cannabis versus Marinol. *J Analyt Toxicol* 23(3):222-4.

Evans, A.T., E.A. Formukong, and F.J. Evans. 1987. Actions of cannabis constituents on enzymes of arachidonate metabolism: anti-inflammatory potential. *Bioch Pharmacol* 36:2035-7.

Evans, F.J. 1991. Cannabinoids: the separation of central from peripheral effects on a structural basis. *Planta Med* 57(Suppl 1):S60-7.

Fairbairn, J.W., and J.T. Pickens. 1981. Activity of cannabis in relation to its delta[1]-trans-tetrahydro-cannabinol content. *British J Pharmacol* 72:401-9.

Falk, A.A., M.T. Hagberg, A.E. Lof, E.M. Wigaeus-Hjelm, and Z.P. Wang. 1990. Uptake, distribution and elimination of alpha-pinene in man after exposure by inhalation. *Scand J Work Envir Health* 16(5):372-8.

Falk-Filipsson, A., A. Löf, M. Hagberg, E.W. Hjelm, and Z. Wang. 1993. *d*-Limonene exposure to humans by inhalation: uptake, distribution, elimination, and effects on the pulmonary function. *J Toxicol Envir Health* 38:77-88.

126 CANNABIS THERAPEUTICS IN HIV/AIDS

Faubert, B.L., and N.E. Kaminski. 2000. AP-1 activity is negatively regulated by cannabinol through inhibition of its protein components, c-fos and c-jun. *J Leukocyte Biol* 67:259-66.

Fenselau, C., and G. Hermann. 1972. Identification of phytosterols in red oil extract of cannabis. *J Forens Sci* 17(2):309-12.

Foletta, V.C., D.H. Segal, and D.R. Cohen. 1998. Transcriptional regulation in the immune system: all roads lead to AP-1. *J Leukocyte Biol* 63:139-52.

Formukong, E.A., A.T. Evans, and F.J. Evans. 1988. Inhibition of the cataleptic effect of tetrahydrocannabinol by other constituents of *Cannabis sativa* L. *J Pharm Pharmacol* 40:132-4.

Franchomme, P. and Pénoël. 1990. *L'aromathérapie exactement*. Limoges, France: Roger Jallois.

Fournier, G., C. Richez-Dumanois, J. Duvezin, J.P. Mathieu, and M. Paris. 1987. Identification of a new chemotype in *Cannabis sativa*: cannabigerol-dominant plants, biogenetic and agronomic prospects. *Planta Med* 53:277-80.

Fuhr, U. 1998. Drug interactions with grapefruit juice. Extent, probable mechanism and clinical relevance. *Drug Safety* 18:251-72.

Gadow, A von, E. Joubert, and C.G. Hansmann. 1997. Comparison of the antioxidant activity of aspalathin with that of other plant phenols of rooibos tea (*Aspalathus linearis*), α-tocopherol, BHT, and BHA. *J Agricult Food Chem* 45:632-8.

Gallily, R., A. Yamin, Y. Waksmann, H. Ovadia, J. Weidenfeld, A. Bar-Joseph, A. Biegon, R. Mechoulam, and E. Shohami. 1997. Protection against septic shock and suppression of tumor necrosis factor alpha and nitric oxide production by dexanabinol (HU-211), a nonpsychotropic cannabinoid. *J Pharm Exper Therap* 283(2): 918-24.

Gerritsen, M.E., W.W. Carley, G.E. Ranges, C.-P. Shen, S.A. Phan, G.F. Ligon, and C.A. Perry. 1995. Flavonoids inhibit cytokine-induced endothelial cell adhesion protein gene expression. *Am J Path* 147:278-92.

Gieringer, D. 1996. Marijuana research: waterpipe study. *MAPS* [Multidisciplinary Association for Psychedelic Studies] *Bull* 6(3):59-66.

Gieringer, D. 2001. NORML study shows vaporizers reduce marijuana smoke toxins. *California NORML Reports* 25(1):2.

Gil, M.L., J. Jimenez, M.A. Ocete, A. Zarzuelo, and M.M. Cabo. 1989. Comparative study of different essential oils of Bupleurum gibraltaricum Lamarck. *Pharmazie* 44(4):284-7.

Gill, E.W., W.D.M. Paton, and R.G. Pertwee. 1970. Preliminary experiments on the chemistry and pharmacology of *Cannabis*. *Nature* 228:134-6.

Gomez, M.A., M.T. Saenz, M.D. Garcia, and M.A. Fernandez. 1999. Study of the topical anti-inflammatory activity of Achillea ageratum on chronic and acute inflammation models. *Zeitscrift fur Naturforsch [C]* 54 (11):937-41.

Greene-McDowelle, D.M., B. Ingber, M.S. Wright, H.J. Zeringue, D. Bhatnagar, and T.E. Cleveland. 1999. The effects of selected cotton-leaf volatiles on growth, development and aflatoxin production of *Aspergillus parasiticus*. *Toxicon* 37: 883-93.

Greenspan, H.C. 1993. The role of reactive oxygen species, antioxidants and phytopharmaceuticals in human immunodeficiency virus activity. *Med Hypoth* 40:85-92.

Grinspoon, L., J.B. Bakalar. 1997. *Marihuana, the forbidden medicine*, revised edition. New Haven, CT: Yale University Press.

Guenther, E. 1948. *The essential oils: Individual essential oils of the plant families.* New York: D. Van Nostrand.

Gwanzura, L., W. McFarland, D. Alexander, R. L. Burke, and D. Katzenstein. 1998. Association between human immunodeficiency virus and herpes simplex virus type 2 seropositivity among male factory workers in Zimbabwe. *J Infect Dis* 177(2): 481-4.

Hammerschmidt, F.J., A.M. Clark, F.M. Soliman, E.S. el-Kashoury, M.M. Abd el-Kawy, and A.M. el-Fishawy. 1993. Chemical composition and antimicrobial activity of essential oils of *Jasonia candicans* and *J. montana. Planta Med* 59(1): 68-70.

Hampson, A.J., M. Grimaldi, J. Axelrod, and D. Wink. 1998. Cannabidiol and $(-)$ Δ^9-tetrahydrocannabinol are neuroprotective antioxidants. *Proc Natl Acad Sci* 95:8268-73.

Hardcastle, I.R., M.G. Rowlands, A.M. Barber, R.M. Grimshaw, M.K. Mohan, B.P. Nutley, and M. Jarman. 1999. Inhibition of protein prenylation by metabolites of limonene. *Biochem Pharmacol* 57:801-9.

Hatoum, N.S., W.M. Davis, M.A. ElSohly, and C.E. Turner. 1981. Cannabichromene and of Δ^9-tetrahydrocannabinol: interactions relative to lethality, hypothermia, and hexobarbital hypnosis. *Gen Pharmacol* 12:357-62.

Herring, A.C., N.E. Kaminski. 1999. Cannabinol-mediated inhibition of nuclear factor-κB, cAMP response element-binding protein, and interleukin-2 secretion by activated thymocytes. *J Pharmacol Exp Therap* 291:1156-63.

Heyser, C.J., R.E. Hampson, and S.A. Deadwyler. 1993. Effects of Δ^9-tetrahydrocannabinol on delayed match to sample performance in rats: alterations in short-term memory associated with changes in task specific firing of hippocampal cells. *J Pharmacol Exp Therap* 264:294-307.

Hollister, L.E. 1974. Structure-activity relationships in man of cannabis constituents, and homologs and metabolites of delta-9-tetrahydrocannabinol. *Pharmacol* 11(1): 3-11.

Hudson, B.J.F., and S.E.O. Mahgoub. 1981. Synergism between phospholipids and naturally-occurring antioxidants in leaf lipids. *J Sci Food Agricult* 32:208-10.

Jones, C.L.A. 1999. Monoterpenes: Essence of a cancer cure. *Nutr Sci News* 4 (4):190.

Kapeghian, J.C., A.B. Jones, J.C. Murphy, M.A. Elsohly, and C.E. Turner. 1983. Effect of cannabichromene on hepatic microsomal enzyme activity in the mouse. *Gen Pharmacol* 14:361-3.

Klein, T.W., C. Newton, and H. Friedman. 1987. Inhibition of natural killer cell function by marijuana components. *J Toxicol Envir Health* 20:321-32.

Klein, T.W., H. Friedman, and S. Specter. 1998. Marijuana, immunity and infection. *J Neuroimmunol* 83:102-5.

Klingeren, B.V., and M.T. Ham. 1976. Antibacterial activity of Δ^9-tetrahydrocannabinol and cannabidiol. *Antonie van Leeuwenhoek* 42:9-12.

Komori, T., R. Fujiwara, M. Tanida, J. Nomura, and M.M. Yokoyama. 1995. Effects of citrus fragrance on immune function and depressive states. *Neuroimmunomod* 2(3):174-80.

Komori, T., R. Fujiwara, M. Tanida, J. Nomura, and M.M. Yokoyama. 1995. Effects of citrus fragrance on immune function and depressive states. *Neuroimmunomod* 2:174-80.

Kovar, K.A., B. Gropper, D. Friess, and H.P. Ammon. 1987. Blood levels of 1,8-cineole and locomotor activity of mice after inhalation and oral administration of rosemary oil. *Planta Med* 53(4):315-8.

Kubena, R.K., and H. Barry. 1972. Stimulus characteristics of marihuana components. *Nature* 235:397-8.

Lawless, J. 1995. *The illustrated encyclopedia of essential oils: the complete guide to the use of oils in aromatherapy and herbalism*. Shaftesbury, Dorset, UK: Element.

Liu, S.L. 1990. [Therapeutic effects of borneol-walnut oil in the treatment of purulent otitis media]. *Chung Hsi I Chieh Ho Tsa Chih* 10(2):93-5, 69.

Lorenzetti, B.B., G.E.P. Souza, S.J. Sarti, D. Santos Filho, and S.H. Ferreira. 1991. Myrcene mimics the peripheral analgesic activity of lemongrass tea. *J Ethnopharmacol* 34:43-8.

Malfait, A.M., R. Gallily, P.F. Sumariwalla, A.S. Malik, E. Andreakos, R. Mechoulam, and M. Feldman. 2000. The nonpsychoactive cannabis constituent cannabidiol is an oral anti-arthritic therapeutic in murine collagen-induced arthritis. *Proc Natl Acad Sci* 97:9561-6.

Malingré, T., H. Hendriks, S. Batterman, R. Bos, and J. Visser. 1975. The essential oil of *Cannabis sativa*. *Planta Med* 28:56-61.

Marcihac, A., N. Dakine, N. Bourhim, V. Guillaume, M. Grino, K. Drieu, and C. Oliver. 1998. Effect of chronic administration of *Ginkgo biloba* extract or kinkgolide on the hypothalamic-pituitary-adrenal axis in the rat. *Life Sci* 62:2329-40.

Martin, L., D.M. Smith, and C.G. Farmilo. 1961. Essential oil from fresh *Cannabis sativa* and its use in identification. *Nature* 191:774-6.

Mathew, R.J., and W.H. Wilson. 1993. Acute changes in cerebral blood flow after smoking marijuana. *Life Sci* 52:757-67.

McPartland, J.M., and P.L. Pruitt. 2000. Benign prostatic hyperplasia treated with saw palmetto: a literature search and an experimental case study. *J Amer Osteopath Assoc* 100(2):89-96.

McPartland, J.M. 1984. Pathogenicity of *Phomopsis ganjae* on *Cannabis sativa* and the fungistatic effect of cannabinoids produced by the host. *Mycopathologia* 87: 149-53.

McPartland, J.M. 1996. Viral hepatitis treated with *Phyllanthus amarus* and milk thistle (*Silybum marianum*): a case report. *Complement Med Internat* 3(2):40-2.

McPartland, J.M. 1997. *Cannabis* as a repellent crop and botanical pesticide. *J Internat Hemp Assoc* 4(2):89-94.

McPartland, J.M., R.C. Clarke, and D.P. Watson. 2000. *Hemp diseases and pests: Management and biological control*. Wallingford: UK. CABI.

McPartland, J.M., and P.P. Pruitt. 1999. Side effects of pharmaceuticals not elicited by comparable herbal medicines: the case of tetrahydrocannabinol and marijuana. *Altern Therap* 5(4):57-62.

McPartland, J.M., and P.P. Pruitt. 1997. Medical marijuana and its use by the immunocompromised. *Altern Therap* 3(3):39-45.

Mechoulam, R., and S. Ben-Shabat. 1999. From gan-zi-gun-nu to anandamide and 2-arachidonoylglycerol: The ongoing story of cannabis. *Nat Prod Rep* 16(2): 131-43.

Mechoulam, R., and Y. Gaoni. 1967. Recent advances in the chemistry of hashish. *Fortschritte der Chemie Organischer Naturstoffe* 25:175-213.

Mechoulam, R., and Y. Gaoni. 1965. Hashish–IV. The isolation and structure of cannabinolic, cannabidiolic, and cannabigerolic acids. *Tetrahedr* 21:1223-9.

Mechoulam, R., Z. Ben-Zvi, A. Shani, H. Zemler, and S. Levy. 1972. Cannabinoids and Cannabis activity. In: *Cannabis and its derivatives*. Paton WDM, Crown J, eds. London: Oxford University Press, pp. 1-13.

Mediavilla, V., and S. Steinemann. 1997. Essential oil of *Cannabis sativa* L. strains. *J Internat Hemp Assoc* 4(2):82-4.

Meier, C., Mediavilla, V. 1998. Factors influencing the yield and the quality of hemp (*Cannabis sativa* L.) essential oil. *J Internat Hemp Assoc* 5(1):16-20.

Merkus, F.W.H.M. 1971. Cannabivarin and tetrahydrocannabivarin, two new constituents of hashish. *Nature* 232:580-1.

Meschler, J.P., and A.C. Howlett. 1999. Thujone exhibits low affinity for cannabinoid receptors but fails to evoke cannabimimetic responses. *Pharmacol Biochem Behav* 62:473-80.

Misner, D.L., and J.M. Sullivan. 1999. Mechanism of cannabinoid effects on long-term potentiation and depression in hippocampal CA1 neurons. *J Neurosci* 19(16): 6795-805.

Miyazawa, M., H. Watanabe, and H. Kameoka. 1997. Inhibition of acetylcholinesterase activity by monoterpenoids with a *p*-methane skeleton. *J Agricult Food Chem* 45:677-9.

Musonda, C.A., and J.K. Chipman. 1998. Quercetin inhibits hydrogen peroxide-induced NF-κB DNA binding activity and DNA damage in HepG2 cells. *Carcinogen* 19:1583-9.

Musty, R.E., I.G. Karniol, I. Shirakawa, N. Takahshi, and E. Knobel. Interactions of Δ^9-THC and cannabinol in man. In: *Pharmacology of marihuana*, MC Braude and S. Szara, eds. Raven Press, NY. Vol. 2:559-63.

Nasel, C., B. Nasel, P. Samec, E. Schindler, and G. Buchbauer. 1994. Functional imaging of effects of fragrances on the human brain after prolonged inhalation. *Chem Senses* 19:359-64.

Nigam, M.C., K.L. Handa, I.C. Nigam, and L. Levi. 1965. Essential oils and their constituents. XXIX. The essential oil of marihuana: composition of the genuine Indian *Cannabis sativa* L. *Canad J Chem* 43:3372-6.

O'Neil, J.D., W.S. Dalton, and R.B. Forney. 1979. The effect of cannabichromene on mean blood pressure, heart rate, and respiration rate responses to tetrahydrocannabinol in the anesthetized rat. *Toxicol Appl Pharmacol* 49:265-70.

Offord, E.A., K. Macé, O. Avanti, and A.M.A. Pfeifer. 1997. Mechanisms involved in the chemoprotective effects of rosemary extract studied in human liver and bronchial cells. *Cancer Lett* 114:275-81.

Ohlsson, A., J.E. Lindgren, A. Wahlen, S. Agurell, L.E. Hollister, and H.K. Gillespie. 1980. Plasma Δ9-tetrahydrocannabinol concentrations and clinical effects after oral and intravenous administration and smoking. *Clin Pharmacol Therap* 28:409-16.

Onawunmi, G.O., W.A. Yisak, and E.O. Ogunlana. 1984. Antibacterial constituents in the essential oil of *Cymbopogon citratus* (DC.) Stapf. *J Ethnopharmacol* 12(3): 279-86.

Ortiz de Urbina, A.V., M.L. Martin, M.J. Montero, A. Moran, and L. San Roman. 1989. Sedating and antipyretic activity of the essential oil of *Calamintha sylvatica* subsp. *ascendens. J Ethnopharmacol* 25(2):165-71.

Paris, R.R., E. Henri, and M. Paris. 1976. Sur les c-flavonoïdes du *Cannabis sativa* L. *Plantes Médicinales et Phytothérapie* 10:144-54.

Parry, E.J. 1918. *The chemistry of essential oils and artificial perfumes.* 2 vols. London: Scott, Greenwood and Son.

Pate, D. 1994. Chemical ecology of cannabis. *J Internat Hemp Assoc* 2:32-7.

Pate, D. 1999. Anandamide structure-activity relationships and mechanisms of action on intraocular pressure in the normotensive rabbit model. PhD thesis, University of Kuopio, Finland, 99 pp.

Perry, N.S., P. J. Houghton, A. Theobald, P. Jenner, and E. K. Perry. 2000. *In-vitro* inhibition of human erythrocyte acetylcholinesterase by salvia lavandulaefolia essential oil and constituent terpenes. *J Pharm Pharmacol* 52(7):895-902.

Perry, N., G. Court, N. Bidet, J. Court, and E. Perry. 1996. European herbs with cholinergic activity: potential in dementia therapy. *Internat J Geriatr Psych* 11: 1063-9.

Petitet, F., B. Jeantaud, A. Imperato, and M.C. Dubroeucq. 1998. Complex pharmacology of natural cannabinoids: evidence for partial agonist activity of Δ^9-tetrahydrocannabinol and antagonist activity of cannabidiol on rat brain cannabinoid receptors. *Life Sci* 63:PL1-6.

Pitts, J.E., J.D. Neal, and T.A. Gough. 1992. Some features of Cannabis plants grown in the United Kingdom from seeds of known origin. *J Pharm Pharmacol* 44(12): 947-51.

Poddar, M.K., and W.L. Dewey. 1980. Effects of cannabinoids on catecholamine uptake and release in hypothalamic and striatal synaptosomes. *J Pharmacol Exper Therap* 214:63-7.

Poirier, J., M.C. Delisle, R. Quirion, et al. 1995. Apolipoprotein E4 allele as a predictor of cholinergic deficits and treatment outcome in Alzheimer's disease. *Proc Natl Acad Sci* 92:12260-4.

Raman, A., U. Weir, and S.F. Bloomfield. 1995. Antimicrobial effects of tea-tree oil and its major components on *Staphylococcus aureus, Staph. epidermidis* and *Propionibacterium acnes. Lett Appl Microbiol* 21(4):242-5.

Rao, V.S.N., A.M.S. Menezes, and G.S.B. Viana. 1990. Effect of myrcene on nociception in mice. *J Pharm Pharmacol* 42:877-8.

Rodríguez de Fonseca, F., P. Rubio, F. Menzaghi, E. Merlo-Pich, J. Rivier, G.F. Koob, and M. Navarro. 1996. Corticotropin-releasing factor (CRF) antagonist (D-Phe[12], Nle[21], C[α]MeLeu[37]) CRF attenuates the acute actions of the highly potent cannabinoid receptor agonist HU-210 on defensive-withdrawal behavior in rats. *J Pharm Exp Therap* 276:56-64.

Rose, J.E., and F.M. Behm. 1994. Inhalation of vapor from black pepper extract reduces smoking withdrawal symptoms. *Drug Alcohol Dep* 34(3):225-9.

Ross, S.A., and M.A. ElSohly. 1996. The volatile oil composition of fresh and air-dried buds of *Cannabis sativa. J Natl Prod* 59:49-51.

Russo, E.B. 2000. *Handbook of psychotropic herbs: A scientific analysis of herbal remedies for psychiatric conditions.* Binghamton, NY: The Haworth Press, Inc.

Russo, E., C.M. Macarah, C.L. Todd, R.S. Medora, and K.K. Parker. 2000. Pharmacology of the essential oil of hemp at 5-HT$_{1A}$ and 5-HT$_{2a}$ receptors. Poster at 41st Annual Meeting of the American Society of Pharmacognosy, July 22-26, Seattle, WA.

Russo, E.B. 2001. Hemp for headache: an in-depth historical and scientific review of cannabis in migraine treatment. *J Cann Therap* 1(2):21-92.

Salgueiro, J.B., P. Ardenghi, M. Dias, M.B.C. Ferreira, I. Izquierdo, and J.H. Medina. 1997. Anxiolytic natural and synthetic flavonoid ligands of the central benzodiazepine receptor have no effect on memory tasks in rats. *Pharmacol Biochem Behav* 58:887-91.

Santos, F.A., and V.S. Rao. 2000. Antiinflammatory and antinociceptive effects of 1,8-cineole a terpenoid oxide present in many plant essential oils. *Phytother Res* 14(4):240-4.

Sauer, M.A., S.M. Rifka, R.L. Hawks, G.B. Cutler, and D.L. Loriaux. 1983. Marijuana: interaction with the estrogen receptor. *J Pharm Exper Therap* 224:404-7.

Setzer, W.N., M.C. Setzer, D.M. Moriarity, R.B. Bates, and W.A. Haber. 1999. Biological activity of the essential oil of *Myrcianthes* sp. *nov.* "black fruit" from Monteverde, Costa Rica. *Planta Med* 65(5):468-9.

Shen, M., and S.A. Thayer. 1999. Δ^9-tetrahydrocannabinol acts as a partial agonist to modulate glutamatergic synaptic transmission between rat hippocampal neurons in culture. *Molec Pharmacol* 55:8-13.

Shimizu, E., Y.P. Tang, C. Rampon, and J.Z. Tsien. 2000. NMDA receptor-dependent synaptic reinforcement as a crucial process for memory consolidation. *Science* 290:1170-73.

Shivers, S.C., C. Newton, H. Friedman, and T.W. Klein. 1994. Δ^9-Tetrahydrocannabinol (THC) modulates IL-1 bioactivity in human monocyte/macrophage cell lines. *Life Sci* 54:1281-9.

Showalter, V.M., D.R. Compton, B.R. Martin, and M.E. Abood. 1996. Evaluation of binding in a transfected cell line expressing a peripheral cannabinoid receptor (CB2): identification of cannabinoid receptor subtype selective ligands. *J Pharm Exper Therap* 278:989-99.

Small, E. 1979. *The Species problem in cannabis. Volume 1: Science.* Ottawa: Corpus Information Services Limited.

Sparacino, C.M., P.A. Hyldburg, and T.J. Hughes. 1990. Chemical and biological analysis of marijuana smoke condensate. *NIDA Res Monogr* 99:121-40.

Tambe, Y., H. Tsujiuchi, G. Honda, Y. Ikeshiro, and S. Tanaka. 1996. Gastric cytoprotection of the non-steroidal anti-inflammatory sesquiterpene, beta-caryophyllene. *Planta Med* 62(5):469-70.

Tashkin, D.P., S. Reiss, B.J. Shapiro, B. Calvarese, J.L. Olsen, and W. Lodge. 1977. Bronchial effects of aerosolized Δ^9-tetrahydrocannabinol in healthy and asthmatic subjects. *Am Rev Resp Dis* 115:57-65.

Thompson, G.R., H. Rosenkrantz, U.H. Schaeppi, and M.C. Braude. 1973. Comparison of acute oral toxicity of cannabinoids in rats, dogs and monkeys. *Toxicol Appl
Pharmacol* 25:363-73.

Tisserand, R., and T. Balacs. 1995. *Essential oil safety: A guide for health care profes-
sionals*. Edinburgh: Churchill Livingstone.

Turner, C.E., M.A. Elsohly, and E.G. Boeren. 1980. Constituents of *Cannabis sativa* L.
XVII. A review of the natural constituents. *J Nat Prod* 43:169-304.

Veszki, P., G. Verzár-Petri, and S. Mészáros. 1980. Comparative phytochemical study
on the cannabinoid composition of the geographical varieties of *Cannabis sativa* L.
under the same condition. *Herba Hungarica* 19:95-102.

Vigushin, D.M., G.K. Poon, A. Boddy, J. English, G.W. Halbert, C. Pagonis, M.
Jarman, and R.C. Coombes. 1998. Phase I and pharmacokinetic study of D-limo-
nene in patients with advanced cancer. Cancer Research Campaign Phase I/II Clinical Trials Committee. *Cancer Chemother Pharmacol* 42(2):111-7.

Walton, R.P. 1938. *Marihuana, America's new drug problem*. J.B. Lippincott Co.,
Philadelphia.

Wang, C., and M.S. Kurzer. 1998. Effects of phytoestrogens on DNA synthesis in
MCF-7 cells in the presence of estradiol or growth factors. *Nutr Cancer* 31:90-100.

Wilt, T.J., A. Ishani, G. Stark, R. MacDonald, J. Lau, and C. Mulrow. 1998. Saw palmetto extracts for treatment of benign prostatic hyperplasia: a systematic review.
J Amer Med Assoc 280(18):1604-9.

Wirth, P.W., E.S. Watson, M. ElSohly, C.E. Turner, and J.C. Murphy. 1980. Anti-inflammatory properties of cannabichromene. *Life Sci* 26:1991-5.

Zuardi, A.W., I. Shirakawa, E. Finkelfarb, and I.G. Karniol. 1982. Action of cannabidiol on the anxiety and other effects produced by Δ^9-THC in normal subjects.
Psychopharmacol 76:245-50.

Zuardi, A.W., S.L. Morais, F.S. Guimarães, and R. Mechoulam. 1995. Antipsychotic
effect of cannabidiol. *J Clin Psychiatr* 56:485-6.

Harm Reduction Associated with Inhalation and Oral Administration of Cannabis and THC

Franjo Grotenhermen

SUMMARY. Inhalation of carcinogenic combustion products associated with smoking is generally regarded as the major health hazard in connection with the medical use of cannabis products. Strategies to reduce respiratory and other adverse events resulting from this common practice include relinquishment of inhalation and replacement by other routes of administration, the use of plants with a high THC content allowing reduction of the amount of smoked plant material, usage of inhalation devices that improve the ratio of THC and tar, and avoidance of the Valsalva maneuver that may cause spontaneous pneumothorax. The major risk associated with oral cannabis use is accidental overdosage, especially in inexperienced users that can be avoided by appropriate dosing procedures. A combination of oral use and inhalation may be meaningful in several indications, decreasing the specific risks of both routes. Preliminary studies using rectal, sublingual and transdermal routes indicate that these alternatives to the two most common forms of ingestion may be utilized medicinally in the future, further reducing the possible risks associated with the administration of cannabis or single cannabinoids. *[Article copies available for a fee from The Haworth Document Delivery Service: 1-800-342-9678. E-mail address: <getinfo@haworthpressinc.com> Website: <http://www.HaworthPress.com> © 2001 by The Haworth Press, Inc. All rights reserved.]*

Franjo Grotenhermen is affiliated with nova-Institut, Goldenbergstraße 2, D-50354 Hürth, Germany (E-mail: franjo-grotenhermen@nova-institut.de).

[Haworth co-indexing entry note]: "Harm Reduction Associated with Inhalation and Oral Administration of Cannabis and THC." Grotenhermen, Franjo. Co-published simultaneously in *Journal of Cannabis Therapeutics* (The Haworth Integrative Healing Press, an imprint of The Haworth Press, Inc.) Vol. 1, No. 3/4, 2001, pp. 133-152; and: *Cannabis Therapeutics in HIV/AIDS* (ed: Ethan Russo) The Haworth Integrative Healing Press, an imprint of The Haworth Press, Inc., 2001, pp. 133-152. Single or multiple copies of this article are available for a fee from The Haworth Document Delivery Service [1-800-342-9678, 9:00 a.m. - 5:00 p.m. (EST). E-mail address: getinfo@haworthpressinc.com].

KEYWORDS. Cannabis, marijuana, THC, cannabinoids, smoking, inhalation, oral use, rectal use, sublingual use, transdermal use, therapeutic use, side effects, health risk, harm reduction, cancer, spontaneous pneumothorax, dosing, overdose, opium, opiates, pharmacokinetics

INTRODUCTION

Major objections to the use of crude cannabis products medicinally are often based not on properties of the natural herb itself, but on the possible adverse health effects resulting from the most prevalent form of application in recreational use: smoking a marijuana cigarette or pipe (Joy et al. 1999; Tashkin 2001). The major advantages of inhalation of cannabis or THC are rapid onset of action and flexible dose titration, making this route of administration very attractive to medical users. Dronabinol is a synonym for the natural ($-$)-trans isomer of delta-9-THC (the pharmacological most active isomer of delta-9-THC that is present in the cannabis plant) when synthesized and manufactured as Marinol®. The oral route is more prone to improper dosing, resulting in unwanted side effects due to overdosage. However, this route may be advantageous if a long duration of drug action is desired. Harm reduction techniques are intended to minimize the health risks associated with different routes of application while maintaining the specific pharmacokinetic advantages.

PHARMACOKINETICS

Depending on method of administration, there are significant differences in absorption and metabolism of THC, attendant effects, time until onset of action, and duration (Table 1).

Pulmonary absorption of cannabis results in maximum THC concentration within about five minutes. THC is detectable in plasma only seconds after the first inhalation. Psychotropic effects commence within seconds to minutes, are maximal after 30 min, and last about 2-3 h. Certain effects may last longer. Thus, Meinck et al. (1989) measured an improvement of some spasticity parameters for more than 12 hours after smoking a cannabis cigarette.

Agurell et al. (1986) noted that only about 20% of the THC present in a marijuana cigarette was absorbed via mainstream smoke when a group of cannabis users inhale in their customary fashion. Thus, most of the THC is lost in side-stream smoke. Effectiveness may be even lower in inexperienced users with a bioavailability below 10%. In experienced users the highest systemic bioavailability measured was 56% (Agurell et al. 1986). Davis et al. (1984) have analyzed smoking characteristics of marijuana cigarettes with a smoking

TABLE 1. Pharmacokinetic comparison of THC application to humans via intravenous, respiratory and oral routes. (Agurell et al. 1986, Azorlosa et al. 1992, Frytak et al. 1984, Wall et al. 1983, Ohlsson et al. 1980, Perez-Reyes et al. 1981, Perez-Reyes et al. 1973)

Parameter	Intravenous	Inhaled	Oral (lipophilic vehicle)
Absorption	100%	10-30 (up to 50)%	> 95%
Systemic bioavailability	100%	10-30 (up to 50)%	10-20%
Psychotropic threshold per kg body weight	0.02 mg/kg	0.06-0.1 mg/kg	0.2-0.3 mg/kg
Psychotropic threshold per individual	1 mg	3-6 mg	ca. 10-20 mg
Maximum plasma concentration at the psychotropic threshold	30-50 ng/ml	30-50 ng/ml	3-5 ng/ml
Dose producing marked intoxication*	2-4 mg	10-20 (up to 50) mg	30-40 (up to 90) mg
Onset of action	within seconds	within seconds	30-60 (up to 120) min
Duration of action**	2-3 (up to 4) h	2-3 (up to 4) h	5-8 (up to 12) h

* Doses producing a marked intoxication vary according to duration of therapy. Longer use may result in the development of tolerance, and higher doses are needed to achieve the similar effects.
** Duration of action varies according to examined effect and especially with oral use according to dose.

machine. When the whole cigarette was consumed in a single puff yielding little side stream smoke, 69% of the THC was preserved in the mainstream smoke, with about 30% lost due to pyrolysis. Smoking a pipe that produces little side stream smoke may also result in high effectiveness, with an average of 45% of THC transferred via the mainstream smoke (Agurell et al. 1986).

After oral ingestion of cannabis, absorption is slow and erratic. Onset of effects is delayed for 30-90 min. Maximum plasma concentrations following 10-15 mg oral THC in sesame oil were noted after 1.75-7 h (Agurell et al. 1986; Brenneisen et al. 1996), usually peaking after about 2 hours. More than one plasma peak may also occur. Compared to inhalation, effects after oral ingestion last longer and fade away more slowly, over 5-8 h, or even longer with very high doses. Duration of action also depends on measured parameters.

Intestinal absorption of THC is increased by application in a lipophilic vehicle. Ohlsson et al. (1980) reported a systemic bioavailability of 6% (±3%) after ingestion of THC in a chocolate cookie. Oral bioavailability was of the order of 10-20% after ingestion of THC in oil capsules (Wall et al. 1983). Therefore, cream or milk can be added to a marijuana tea, or a recipe with plenty of butter may be used if the drug is baked in confections. Δ^9-THC may be degraded by the acid of the stomach and in the gut. Several competing reactions occur at low pH, among them isomerization to Δ^8-THC and protonation of the oxygen in the pyran ring, causing ring cleavage to substituted cannabidiols (Agurell et al. 1986). In lipophilic vehicles, such as in the case of Marinol® capsules, where THC is dissolved in sesame oil, at least 95% of THC is absorbed from the gastrointestinal tract (Wall et al. 1983). Due to an extensive first-pass liver metabolism and pre-systemic elimination in the gut, with oral application systemic bioavailability is only 10-20% (Agurell et al. 1986).

In the cannabis plant, about 95% of Δ^9-THC is present as one of two pharmacologically inactive acid forms, the Δ^9-THC carboxylic acids (THCA) (Turner et al. 1980). Natural cannabinoids must be decarboxylated before ingestion, since the corresponding neutral phenolic forms of THC produce most biological effects. The simplest and fastest way to achieve this is through heating (smoking, baking, cooking). Neutral phenols are responsible for the known pharmacological effects of dronabinol. Five minutes of heating to 200-210°C has been determined as the optimal condition for complete decarboxylation of THCA without oxidation to cannabinol (Brenneisen 1984). In cannabis smoking, where temperatures of 600°C are achieved, only a few seconds of combustion are apparently sufficient for decarboxylation.

INHALATION OR ORAL APPLICATION

Cannabis and THC can both be administered by various routes. Inhalation and oral use are the most frequent ways to ingest the drug, each demonstrating particular advantages and disadvantages. The advantage of oral intake is its more constant and prolonged activity, for example, in the prevention of nocturnal spasms in multiple sclerosis, or decreasing intraocular pressure for several hours. Its disadvantage is possible overdosage, especially with cannabis preparations of unknown THC content.

The major advantages of inhalation are fast onset of action and easy titration of dose. These are preferable in acute disorders that demand a fast effect, such as rapidly treating a migraine attack, or combating breakthrough pain. Inhalation is also superior to ingestion by mouth in nausea and vomiting, where it may be difficult to take pills or other oral preparations. The disadvantage of smoking is potential damage to the respiratory tract.

RISKS OF SMOKING

More than 200 combustion products have been found in marijuana smoke (Sparacino et al. 1990), and many are known to be toxic to tissues of the respiratory and upper intestinal tract. Aside from the nicotine content, cannabis smoke is qualitatively similar to that of tobacco (Tashkin 2001). Benzo[α]anthracene and benzo[α]pyrene, two highly procarcinogenic polycyclic aromatic hydrocarbons (PAHs) are present in 25-75% higher concentrations in the tar from cannabis as compared to tobacco (Lee et al. 1976). The deposition of PAHs is amplified approximately 4 times by a higher tar yield of unfiltered marijuana cigarettes compared to filter-tipped tobacco cigarettes, and a longer breathholding time with marijuana (Wu et al. 1988). A 4-fold longer breathholding results in a 40% greater deposition of tar in the respiratory tract (Wu et al. 1988).

Whether this higher tar yield from cannabis smoke leads to a fourfold stronger damage of the mucosa compared to smoking the same amount of tobacco is unclear. A fourfold increase may be regarded as the worst-case scenario, whereby smoking half a cannabis cigarette (about 0.4 grams of cannabis) would damage the mucosa to a similar degree as two tobacco cigarettes (see Figure 1). Histopathological alterations of the airways associated with smoking may lead to chronic bronchitis and, hypothetically, eventually to chronic

FIGURE 1. Assumed risk associated with smoking herbal cannabis vs. THC content (as % of the dried plant material) corresponding to that caused by tobacco cigarettes. The worst-case scenario is assumed, that smoking a certain amount of cannabis increases the risk of respiratory cancer and other damage 4 times higher than smoking the same amount of tobacco (see text). The risk of 0.2 grams of cannabis corresponded to 1 tobacco cigarette. Depending on THC content 0.2 grams of cannabis contain 4 mg (2% THC), 10 mg (5% THC), 20 mg (10% THC) or 40 mg THC (20% THC). About 4 puffs are needed to smoke 0.2 grams of cannabis (see Table 2).

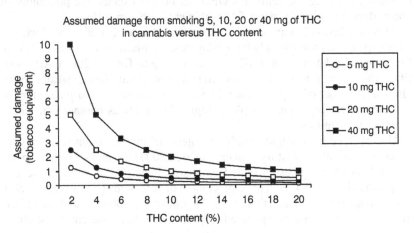

Assumed damage from smoking 5, 10, 20 or 40 mg of THC in cannabis versus THC content

obstructive pulmonary disease (COPD). Epidemiological and experimental data with regard to COPD are conflicting, however. Progressive airways narrowing in COPD can be detected by an accelerated decline in the forced expiratory volume in one second (FEV_1) and by a decreased ratio of FEV_1 to forced vital capacity (FVC). In a study by Bloom et al. (1987), marijuana smokers showed significant lower values for the FEV_1/ FVC ratio than nonsmokers and tobacco smokers. The prevalence of respiratory symptoms was increased. A 6-yr follow-up study with 1802 subjects demonstrated a significant reduction in FEV_1, and FEV_1/FVC in previous marijuana users but not in current users (Sherrill et al. 1991).

In contrast to these findings, a study by Tashkin et al. (1987) comparing marijuana smokers, tobacco smokers, smokers of both tobacco and marijuana, and nonsmokers, did not reveal any association between heavy use of marijuana for more than 15 years and resulting decrements in pulmonary function. None of the values of the applied sensitive measures was different from the average values observed in nonsmokers. In a second study, Tashkin et al. (1997) once more failed to find any association between marijuana use and lung function abnormality. FEV_1 was measured in 131 heavy, habitual smokers of marijuana alone, 112 smokers of marijuana plus tobacco, 65 regular smokers of tobacco alone, and 86 nonsmokers of either substance and in 255 subjects on up to six additional occasions over a period of 8 years. In neither men nor women was marijuana smoking associated with greater declines in FEV_1 than nonsmoking, nor was an additive effect of marijuana and tobacco noted, nor a significant relationship found between the number of marijuana cigarettes smoked per day and the rate of decline in FEV_1. In comparison, tobacco smoking was associated with greater annual rates of decline in lung function than nonsmoking. The authors concluded that "these findings do not support an association between regular marijuana smoking and chronic COPD but do not exclude the possibility of other adverse respiratory effects" (Tashkin et al. 1997, p. 141).

This conclusion is supported by experimental animal studies in which rats were exposed to progressively increasing doses of marijuana or tobacco smoke for six months (Huber et al. 1987, cited according to Tashkin 2001). After sacrifice, the lungs of the tobacco-exposed rats showed morphological and physiological evidence of emphysema, while the rats exposed to marijuana showed no detectable morphologic or physiologic abnormalities compared to unexposed control animals.

However, epidemiological studies suggest that marijuana smoking may increase the risk of respiratory cancer (Tashkin 2001). Bronchial wall biopsies in smokers of marijuana revealed extensive hyperplastic, metaplastic and dysplastic changes believed to be precursors of carcinoma (Fligiel et al. 1997). The damage was similar to that of regular smokers of tobacco, and the effects of marijuana and tobacco appeared to be additive. In a case-control study of

173 patients with newly diagnosed squamous cell carcinoma of the head and neck and 176 cancer-free matched controls, marijuana use was associated with a more than twofold increased risk of head and neck cancer and a dose-response relationship was found (Zhang et al. 1999).

Damage to the mucosa by cannabis smoking, and the presence of pathogens in the plant material may increase the risk of infections, and are of special concern in immunocompromised patients. Cannabis smoke may harbor bacteria and fungi such as *Aspergillus, Mucor* and *Fusarium* species, *Klebsiella pneumoniae, Enterobacter cloacae*, group D *Streptococcus*, some *Bacillus* species and others (for a review see: McPartland 2001).

Performance of the Valsalva maneuver may cause barotrauma to the lung and increase the risk for spontaneous pneumothorax and pneumomediastinum (Feldmann et al. 1993; Miller et al. 1972). Cannabis smokers may typically perform the Valsalva maneuver against a closed glottis after deep inhalation to increase intrathoracic pressure and absorption rate of THC.

HARM REDUCTION WITH INHALATION

The major strategies to reduce the risks of smoking are:

- *The use of cannabis strains with high THC content.* The average concentration of Δ^9-THC in marijuana confiscated in the USA was 4.2% in 1997 (ElSohly et al. 2000). Currently, high-grade cannabis with THC concentrations of 10-20% in the dried flowers is available, reducing the amount necessary for medicinal use and potential damage to the mucosa (see Figure 1). If a strain with a THC content of 10% is used, one puff provides about 5 mg THC (see Table 2). In studies with HIV/AIDS patients, daily doses of 2.5-20 mg have been used to treat anorexia and cachexia, or nausea and vomiting. In a long-term study by Beal et al. (1997) patients received dronabinol orally 2.5 mg once or twice daily to effectively treat anorexia and cachexia in HIV/AIDS. Conant et al. (1991) applied between 2.5 mg dronabinol twice daily and 5 mg three times a day. In a small study by Gorter et al. (1992) participants received between 2×2.5 mg and 4×5 mg dronabinol. Abrams et al. (2000) used smoked cannabis (3.95% THC) and oral dronabinol (3×2.5 mg). Due to the development of some tolerance doses are often increased up to 20 mg with long duration of therapy (personal communications from several physicians), equivalent to one quarter of a marijuana cigarette containing 800 mg of cannabis of 10% THC.
- *The use of pure cannabis.* Sometimes cannabis is smoked together with tobacco or other dried herbs. This procedure should be avoided to minimize the inhalation of smoke from burnt plant material.

- *The use of pipes.* Pipes are superior to cigarettes in some situations in that they easily allow the patient to smoke small amounts of pure high-grade cannabis. The percentage of tars in the smoke is reduced by condensation on the pipe walls. Pipes should be cleaned frequently. Water pipes are inferior to cigarettes and should be avoided (see below).

- *The use of cannabis that is free of natural contaminants and adulterants.* Only disease-free cannabis should be harvested and air-dried. Gross infection with pathogens is easily detectable. Ungerleider et al. (1982) proposed two methods of sterilization: gas-sterilization in a mix of 12% ethylene oxide and 88% dichlorodifluoromethane, and sterilization with Cobalt 60 irradiation. Neither method reduced THC content. Baking plant material in home ovens at 150°C for five minutes kills spores of *Aspergillus fumigatus, A. flavus* and *A. niger* without reducing THC content (McPartland 2001).

- *The use of inhalation devices that reduce output of tars.* Gieringer tested vaporizers that heat marijuana to 180-190°C vaporizing THC below the burning point of cellulose and other plant material. The production of polycyclic hydrocarbons was reduced. The best vaporizer delivered 10 parts of tar to one part of cannabinoids, while in contrast, cannabis cigarettes yielded a ratio of 13:1 (average), and water pipes an average of 27:1 (cited in McPartland 2001). Thus, the best vaporizers achieved a performance ratio about 25% higher than the unfiltered cannabis cigarette, while water pipes were less favorable than cigarettes. The use of a filter in a cannabis cigarette was not advantageous since it not only filtered the tars, but also the cannabinoids. Indeed, the performance ratio was decreased by about 30% compared to the unfiltered cigarette (Gieringer 2000). In a new study Gieringer (2001) was able to demonstrate that combustion products were substantially reduced with another vaporizer. The device used produced THC at a temperature of 185°C while completely eliminating benzene, toluene and naphthalene. Significant amounts of benzene began to appear at temperatures of 200°C, while combustion occurred around 230°C or above. Traces of THC were in evidence as low as 140°C. Carbon monoxide and tars were both qualitatively reduced by the vaporizer, but were not quantified in this study. However, a significant reduction of polycyclic aromatic hydrocarbons was assumed since vaporized cannabis emitted a thin gray vapor and the plant material was left with a green to greenish-brown "toasted" appearance, whereas the combusted sample produced thick smoke and turned to ash.

- *Omission of the Valsalva maneuver and prolonged breathholding.* Several techniques are used to enhance THC absorption in the lungs including the Valsalva maneuver and prolonged breathholding. The first may cause barotrauma to the lung, while the second increases the deposition of tars (see above). According to two quantitative studies (Tashkin et al. 1991; Azorlosa et al. 1995) that correlated breathholding and resulting effects, longer breathholding enhanced THC effects, thus, confirming in part a common behavior of cannabis smokers. However, extended breathholding did not seem to further maximize absorption. Azorlosa et al. (1995) compared breathholding of 0, 10 and 20 seconds in seven subjects who took 10 puffs of cannabis containing 1.75 or 3.55% THC (Figure 2). Maximum THC plasma concentrations after smoking were 61.2, 146.6, and 130.6 ng/ml with the more potent cigarettes. While THC concentrations significantly increased between the 0 sec and the 10 sec conditions, there was no further increase in plasma concentrations by prolonging breathholding from 10 to 20 sec. Thus, prolonged breathholding may increase the amount of deposited tar without increasing THC absorption.

• *Combination of oral use and inhalation.* In several indications, a combined regime of a basic oral medication with cannabis or THC and a demand inhaled medication may be useful to reduce risks from smoking and overdosage with oral administration. Similar regimes are routine with opiates to treat chronic and breakthrough pain (Stevens and Ghazi 2000).

RISKS OF ORAL USAGE

Responsiveness to the action of THC shows a high inter-individual variation. 10 mg of oral THC will not consistently result in psychic alterations, but in some persons even 2.5 mg produce recognizable effects. In a study by Chesher et al. (1990) of a healthy population dosed orally with 5 mg THC, no difference was found to placebo controls as to the subjective level of intoxication. Doses of 10 and 15 mg THC caused slight differences compared to the placebo, and a dose of 20 mg, finally, caused marked differences in subjective perception. In a clinical study by Beal et al. (1995) in AIDS patients some patients experienced mostly mild to moderate side effects (euphoria, dizziness) with 2.5 mg dronabinol twice daily. Lucas and Laszlo (1980) found pronounced psychotropic reactions (anxiety, marked visual distortions) in patients undergoing cancer chemotherapy that had received 15 mg THC/m^2 (square meter of body surface), which corresponds to about 25 mg THC in an average adult person of 1.7 m^2 body surface area. A reduction to 5 mg THC/m^2, about 7.5-10 mg THC, produced only mild reactions. In a study by Frytak et al. (1979) in cancer patients receiving 15 mg dronabinol three times a day as an antiemetic, 52% reported a "high." Brenneisen et al. (1996) administered single oral doses of 10 or 15 mg THC to two patients. Physiologic parameters (heart rate) and psychological parameters (concentration, mood) were not modified by the administration.

TABLE 2. Dosing-scheme for cannabis taken orally and smoked

Amount of cannabis taken	THC content in herbal cannabis		
	2% THC	5% THC	10% THC
oral			
0.05 g	1 mg THC	2.5 mg THC	5 mg THC
0.1 g	2 mg THC	5 mg THC	10 mg THC
0.2 g	4 mg THC	10 mg THC	20 mg THC
0.5 g	10 mg THC	25 mg THC	50 mg THC
smoking*			
1 puff (0.05 g)	1 mg THC	2.5 mg THC	5 mg THC
2 puffs (0.10 g)	2 mg THC	5 mg THC	10 mg THC
4 puffs (0.20 g)	4 mg THC	10 mg THC	20 mg THC
8 puffs (0.40 g)	8 mg THC	20 mg THC	40 mg THC
16 puffs (0.80 g)	16 mg THC	40 mg THC	80 mg THC

* Ingested THC was calculated according to the formula: x = amount of cannabis/100 by THC content. It was assumed that an average of 50 mg of cannabis are smoked with one puff, calculated from the following data. Marijuana cigarettes provided by the U.S. National Institute of Drug Abuse (NIDA) weigh about 800 mg (Azorlosa et al. 1992, Azorlosa et al. 1995). Perez-Reyes et al. (1981) noticed that about 24 puffs were necessary to smoke a low-dose NIDA marijuana cigarette, corresponding to 33 mg of cannabis per puff. Liguori et al. (1998) used a smoking regime with 64 mg marijuana per puff. It should be noted that THC becomes concentrated in the uncombusted parts of a cigarette so that the first puffs yield a little less THC than the later (Tashkin et al. 1991).

Additionally, there may be an intra-individual variance of THC absorption, especially if the drug is taken under different conditions. Intestinal absorption and degradation of THC may depend on several factors. As with opioids, onset of action might depend on the presence or absence of food. Immediate release oral opioid preparations are known to require about 30 minutes to onset of analgesic action taken on an empty stomach, but onset of action may be delayed when taken on a full stomach (Stevens and Ghazi 2000).

Due to the delayed onset of action, oral cannabis products may be difficult to dose precisely, resulting in either overdosage or underdosage, an observation often reported by physicians of the nineteenth century (Fankhauser 2001).

HARM REDUCTION WITH ORAL USE

The major risk associated with oral cannabis use is overdosing. To achieve appropriate dosing two principles should be followed:

FIGURE 2. Average plasma THC levels (ng/ml) in seven healthy young males following ten puffs from a cannabis cigarette containing 1.75 or 3.55% THC with a breathholding duration of 0, 10, and 20 seconds immediately after smoking (drawn according to data from Azorlosa et al. 1995).

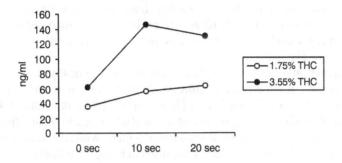

- Ascertainment of optimal individual dose by slowly increasing doses.
- Intake of the medication under the consistent conditions, especially with regard to vehicle and filling of the stomach.
- Subsequent administration of supplemental doses by inhalation.

If possible, slowly increasing doses should be applied in a titrated fashion to avoid undesirable side effects on psyche and circulation. Starting doses are 2 × 2.5 mg or 2 × 5.0 mg of dronabinol per day. Dosages may be increased up to several units of 10 mg daily. In AIDS wasting and HIV related nausea and vomiting 5-20 mg THC daily are usually sufficient (Beal et al. 1995; Beal et al. 1997; Gorter et al. 1992; Abrams et al. 2000). If natural cannabis products of unknown THC content are used orally, the patient should begin with about 0.05-0.1 g of the drug (for cannabis with an average THC content of 5% this corresponds to 2.5-5 mg THC, see Table 2).

If possible, the THC content should be determined in a laboratory. If this is not possible, a store of cannabis sufficient for several weeks should be secured so that a constant quality is ensured. In a study by Fairbairn et al. (1976) the THC content of marijuana only decreased by 7% within 47 weeks with dry storage in the dark at 5°C, and by 13% at a temperature of 20°C.

To achieve reproducible effects, cannabis or THC should always be ingested under similar conditions with regard to food intake, e.g., one hour before a meal. If natural cannabis preparations are used, doses should be weighed carefully and taken with the same carrier, e.g., tea with half a gram of dried cannabis flowers in half a liter of water and some cream.

As with opiates, some side effects may decrease within a period of days or weeks, thereby increasing the acceptance of the drug. Prolonged THC ingestion causes tolerance to orthostatic hypotension, tachycardia and psychological effects (Benowitz and Jones, 1975), so that daily doses of more than 50 mg THC may sometimes be taken without significant undesirable psychic or physical side effects (Holdcroft et al. 1997). Heavy chronic users in western societies may smoke five to ten cannabis cigarettes per day, thus well tolerating daily doses of 100 mg THC and more. In a sample analyzed by Solowij (1991) mean weekly consumption was 766 mg of THC, with a range from 30-2400 mg THC.

Tolerance may also arise with respect to therapeutically desired effects (e.g., decrease of intraocular pressure, analgesia), and require increased doses (Jones et al. 1981). O'Shaughnessy (1839) reported development of tolerance in connection with the medical use of a cannabis tincture in rheumatism: Two of three treated patients showed good improvement, while the third patient did not respond to the drug. He finally admitted to being a habitual user.

Duration of tolerance to THC differs depending on effect. In mice hypothermia, depression of intestinal motility and spontaneous locomotor activity were investigated (Anderson et al. 1975). Normal hypothermic responses returned after 12 dose-free days and baseline locomotor activity returned within 4 days. Tolerance to the depressant effect on intestinal motility still persisted after 19 dose-free days. According to self-reports of patients to the author, tolerance may remain for some weeks to months after stopping the drug.

TREATMENT OF ACCIDENTAL OVERDOSE

Ingestion of cannabis and THC may result in unwanted effects on the circulatory system (increased heart rate, changes of blood pressure) and psychological effects such as an acute panic reaction and hallucinatory experiences (Hall and Solowij, 1998).

Tachycardia may be undesirable in persons suffering from coronary heart disease. It seems to be caused by sympathetic stimulation and can be treated by beta-blockers. Perez-Reyes et al. (1973) used propranolol infused at a rate of 0.5 mg per minute for 6 minutes to block the acceleration of heart rate following oral administration of 35 mg THC in different vehicles. The psychological effect was not altered. Thus, it may be also possible to use beta-blockers as prophylactic agents in individuals with heart disease without influencing other specific effects of THC, including therapeutic actions. In case of orthostatic hypotension or syncope, the patient should lie down with the legs elevated.

"Talking the patient down" may treat dysphoric states. If this proves insufficient, intravenous diazepam (5-10 mg) may be administered (Perez-Reyes et al. 1973).

ALTERNATIVE FORMS OF DELIVERY

Many other forms of application have been tested experimentally, decreasing the time until onset of action compared to oral use and leading to more reliable reproduction of effects. Some routes may be promising in the future.

Sublingual: At the 2000 Meeting of the International Cannabinoid Research Society a British group presented data on studies performed with three different sublingual cannabis extracts (Guy et al. 2000). They had been administered to six healthy volunteers receiving up to 20 mg THC. The group reported that sublingual administration of cannabis extract resulted in relatively fast effects and was well tolerated. No quantitative data on bioavailability are yet available.

Rectal: A few studies have been conducted with rectal THC preparations (Mattes et al. 1994; Brenneisen et al. 1996). Bioavailability strongly differed depending on suppository formulations. Among the formulations containing several polar esters of Δ^9-THC in various suppository bases, Δ^9-THC-hemisuccinate in Witepsol H15 showed the highest bioavailability (ElSohly et al. 1991), about as twice as high as with oral administration in man (Brenneisen et al. 1996).

The author of this article is aware of experiments by several cannabis users, who rectally self-administered natural cannabis preparations. In one example, dried milled cannabis flowers were cooked in cocoa butter for one hour. After cooling, suppositories were formed. The effect was noticeable within about ten minutes. No scientific data are available in this regard. These personal experiences contrast with experimental data according to which unchanged delta-9-THC is not bioavailable by the rectal route (Perlin et al. 1985; ElSohly et al. 1991).

In a study by ElSohly et al. (1991) with various esters of THC in both lipophilic and hydrophilic suppository bases (Witepsol H15 and polyethylene glycol), no delta 9-THC or its metabolites were detected in the blood samples using the Witepsol H15 with the exception of the hemisuccinate ester. Using polyethylene glycol, only low levels of delta 9-THC and its metabolites were detected in blood for all esters tested.

Transdermal: The scientific literature provides little specific information on the transdermal uptake of THC from topically applied preparations. There are only two experimental studies investigating the skin permeation behavior of THC (Touitou and Fabin 1988; Touitou et al. 1988). These investigations were designed to develop an effective transdermal delivery system for THC, an antiemetic in patients receiving cancer chemotherapy. Researchers in this study used Δ^8-THC since this molecule is more stable than the Δ^9-THC.

Generally, the human skin is well protected against penetration by external substances. Many topically applied substances attain a systemic bioavailability of only a few percent (Hadgraft 1996). The main barrier to penetration is the cornified layer of the stratum corneum. There is evidence that only a small fraction of strongly lipophilic substances, such as THC, overcome the hydrophilic phases of the intercellular space between the cells of the stratum corneum (Bast 1997).

However, the uptake of compounds via the skin can be influenced by the presence of other compounds in the matrix. Penetration enhancers may disrupt the stratum corneum lipids, interact with intercellular proteins, or improve the partitioning of a compound. These may include synthetic chemicals such as dimethylsulfoxide (DMSO), surfactants, and certain unsaturated fatty acids, e.g., oleic acid.

The research by Touitou et al. (1988) showed that the permeability coefficient of Δ^8-THC was significantly enhanced by water and by oleic acid in propylene glycol and ethanol (PG-EtOH). Significant THC concentrations in the blood of rats treated with formulations containing 26.5 mg/g THC on the skin were measured. The permeability coefficient of THC was increased 6 times by 3% oleic acid in PG-EtOH solutions and 14 times by 3% oleic acid in PG-EtOH-H_2O solutions (Touitou and Fabin 1988).

An Albany College of Pharmacy research team was awarded a $361,000 three-year grant in January 2000 by the American Cancer Society to study whether cannabinoids can be absorbed effectively through the skin (Gormeley 2000). The research is intended to develop a cannabinoid patch for therapeutic use and is expected to require several years for completion.

The US Patent and Trademark Office granted a patent for a "Cannabinoid patch and method for cannabis transdermal delivery" on September 5, 2000 (United States Patent 6,113,940). The patent describes a trial in two subjects who received 0.2 g of cannabis oil in a carrier (DMSO). The patch was applied to the underside of the wrist of two human subjects. According to the patents, subjective THC effects were noted within ten minutes and lasted four to six hours.

SOME COMPARISONS TO OPIUM OPIATES

There are some parallels between opiates and cannabinoids with regard to mechanism of action and indications (Vaughan and Christie 2001), which shall be discussed in brief, mainly with regard to side effects and routes of administration.

Cannabis (*Cannabis sativa* L.) and opium (*Papaver somniferum* L.) are used recreationally, most often by inhaling the smoke of the burnt plant material. In contrast to cannabis, the illegal use of single opium compounds (natural opiates and their derivatives) are more common today than the use of whole plant preparations. As with cannabis, the specific chronic health effects associated with the use of illegal opiates and opioids largely depend on the route of application.

While smoking is the major route of application for cannabis, it is injection into the blood vessels for opiates. Injection may result in local injury and inflammation, and in the transmission of hepatitis C and HIV through contaminated needles. The chronic use of non-injected opiates seems to cause only minor health effects (Hall et al. 1999). It is remarkable to note that smoking is generally regarded as a minor health hazard in context with opiates (Hall et al. 1999) but seems to be of greater concern in context with cannabis (Joy et al. 1999).

Opium contains about 25 alkaloids. As with cannabis there is one most prominent ingredient. Morphine is present in the plant with 10-15% of dry plant weight. However, there are other pharmacologically potent alkaloids in relevant concentrations, particularly codeine (1%-3%), noscapine (4%-8%), and papaverine (1%-3%).

In addition to the medical use of single natural constituents of opium (morphine, codeine, noscapine), doctors in many countries (e.g., Germany) may also prescribe whole opium preparations. The effects of opium differ qualitatively from that of morphine. Due to the presence of other alkaloids, especially papaverine, opium causes an atonic constipation, in contrast to a spastic constipation with morphine (Mutschler 1996). The difference between whole cannabis and single dronabinol remains to be elucidated, and it is unclear whether this difference is less prominent than between opium and morphine (see McPartland and Russo 2001 in this issue).

There are major differences between the pharmacokinetics of opiates and cannabinoids. To achieve a fast onset of action, hydrophilic opiates may be given intravenously. But the intravenous application of THC is complicated by its lipophilic properties. Even oral opiates have a faster onset than oral cannabinoids (30 min versus 30-90 min) and show a more constant and reliable absorption (Cleary 1997). In contrast to the situation with opiates, there is currently no good available alternative to the inhalation of cannabis or cannabinoids if a fast onset of action is required. The sublingual application of cannabis preparations currently under investigation in clinical studies in the United Kingdom seems to be a promising route.

PRINCIPLES OF HARM REDUCTION WITH CANNABIS

Natural cannabis is usually inhaled. However, this route of administration is often used even if the advantages over oral application are not really of relevance to achieve optimal therapeutic benefits. In cases where inhalation is the best way to administer cannabis or single cannabinoids, techniques designed to reduce risks to the mucosa should be applied. Harm reduction with regard to the medical use of cannabis may include the following strategies:

- Relinquishment of inhalation and replacement by other routes of administration if possible, or combination of several routes.
- Minimization of damage to the respiratory tract with appropriate techniques including the use of cannabis with high THC content, inhalation with vaporizers, avoidance of the Valsalva maneuver and prolonged breath holding over 10 sec.
- Avoidance of accidental over-dosing through thorough dosing procedures with oral ingestion.
- Development and improvement of non-smoked, parenteral application forms, including the rectal, sublingual, and transdermal route.

Taken together these maxims allow reduction in the risks associated with the oral and inhalation routes of administration to a tolerable degree.

Since many physicians reject the concept of smoking medication on principle, it may be helpful to look at this controversial topic in a broader context. To ingest 20 mg of THC, 0.2 g of cannabis (or a quarter of a cigarette) with a THC content of 10% has to be smoked (see Figure 1). Even if a 4-fold health risk potential for cannabis smoke compared to tobacco smoke is assumed, this would result in an equivalent of the respiratory risks associated with smoking one tobacco cigarette a day.

The principle *nihil nocere* ("do no harm"), and the association with recreational usage of cannabis may be regarded as the two major reasons for dismissing smoking. This rejection may evoke a more emotional than scientific attitude towards this question. It should be noted that other accepted routes of administration for many drugs designed to achieve a rapid onset of action are associated with multiple risks, even fatal ones, and various drugs also damage the mucosa. Intravenous or intramuscular application of a drug may harm surrounding tissues and in some cases may produce severe damage. Oral administration of various drugs adversely affects the mucosa of the intestinal tract, among them widely used non-steroidal anti-inflammatory drugs (NSAIDs), such as indomethacin and acetylsalicylic acid. We customarily accept relatively high medical risks, as with intrathecal administration of opioids, if the anticipated benefits outweigh those drawbacks. The inhalation of a limited amount of combustion products with smoked cannabis may be regarded as a rather low and acceptable risk as well, if the benefit for a patient is high.

REFERENCES

Abrams, D.I., R.J. Leiser, S.B. Shade, J. Hilton, and T. Elbeik. 2000. Short-term effects of cannabinoids on HIV-1 viral load. Poster presented at the 13th International AIDS Conference in Durban/South Africa, 13th of July 2000.

Anderson, P.F., D.M. Jackson, G.B. Chesher, and R. Malor. 1975. Tolerance to the effect of delta-9-tetrahydrocannabinol in mice on intestinal motility, temperature and locomotor activity. *Psychopharmacologia* 43(1):31-36.

Azorlosa, J.L., M.K. Greenwald, and M.L. Stitzer. 1995. Marijuana smoking: effects of varying puff volume and breathhold duration. *J Pharmacol Exp Ther* 272(2): 560-569.

Bast, G. E. 1997. Influence of solubility and permeant size on absorption and metabolism of xenobiotics in rabbit skin. *Hum Exp Toxicol* 16:435-440.

Beal, J.E., R. Olson, L. Laubenstein, J.O. Morales, P. Bellman, B. Yangco, L. Lefkowitz, T.F. Plasse, and K.V. Shepard. 1995. Dronabinol as a treatment for anorexia associated with weight loss in patients with AIDS. *J Pain Symptom Manag* 10(2):89-97.

Beal, J.E., R. Olson, L. Lefkowitz, L. Laubenstein, P. Bellman, B. Yangco, J.O. Morales, R. Murphy, W. Powderly, T.F. Plasse, K.W. Mosdell, and K.V. Shepard. 1997. Long-term efficacy and safety of dronabinol for acquired immunodeficiency syndrome-associated anorexia. *J Pain Symptom Manag* 14(1):7-14.

Benowitz, N.L., and R.T. Jones. 1975. Cardiovascular effects of prolonged delta-9-tetrahydrocannabinol ingestion. *Clin Pharmacol Ther* 18(3):287-297.

Bloom, J.W., W.T. Kaltenborn, P. Paoletti, A. Camilli, and M.D. Lebowitz. 1987. Respiratory effects of non-tobacco cigarettes. *Br Med J* 295:1516-1518.

Brenneisen R. 1984. Psychotrope Drogen. II. Bestimmung der Cannabinoide in *Cannabis sativa* L. und in Cannabisprodukten mittels Hochdruckflüssigkeitschromatographie (HPLC). *Pharm Acta Helv* 59(9-10):247-259.

Brenneisen, R., A. Egli, M.A. ElSohly, V. Henn, and Y. Spiess. 1996. The effect of orally and rectally administered Δ9-tetrahydrocannabinol on spasticity: a pilot study with 2 patients. *Int J Clin Pharmacol Ther* 34(10):446-452.

Chesher, G.B., K.D. Bird, D.M. Jackson, A. Perrignon, and G.A. Starmer. 1990. The effects of orally administered delta 9-tetrahydrocannabinol in man on mood and performance measures: a dose-response study. *Pharmacol Biochem Behav* 35(4): 861-864.

Cleary, J.F. 1997. Pharmacokinetic and pharmacodynamic issues in the treatment of breakthrough pain. *Semin Oncol* 24(5 Suppl 16):13-19.

Conant, M., D. Roy, K.V. Shepard, and T.F. Plasse. 1991. Dronabinol enhances appetite and controls weight loss in HIV patients. *Proc Annu Meet Am Soc Clin Oncol* 10:A9.

Davis, K.H., I.A. McDaniel, L.W. Cardwell, and P.L. Moody. 1984. Some smoking characteristics of marijuana cigarettes. In: Agurell, S., W.L. Dewey, and R.E. Willette. eds. *The cannabinoids: Chemical, pharmacologic, and therapeutic aspects*. New York: Academic Press, pp. 97-109.

ElSohly, M.A., S.A. Ross, Z. Mehmedic, R. Arafat, B. Yi, and B.F. Banahan, 3rd. 2000. Potency trends of delta 9-THC and other cannabinoids in confiscated marijuana from 1980-1997. *J Forensic Sci* 45(1):24-30.

Elsohly, M.A., T.L. Little, Jr., A. Hikal, E. Harland, D.F. Stanford, and L. Walker. 1991. Rectal bioavailability of delta-9-tetrahydrocannabinol from various esters. *Pharmacol Biochem Behav* 40(3):497-502.

Fairbairn, J.W., J.A. Liebmann, and M.G. Rowan. 1976. The stability of cannabis and its preparations on storage. *J Pharm Pharmacol* 28(1):1-7.

Feldman, A., J.T. Sullivan, M.A. Passero, and D.C. Lewis. 1993. Pneumothorax in polysubstance abusing marijuana and tobacco smokers: 3 cases. *J Subst Abuse* 5(2):183-186.

Fligiel, S.E.G., M.D. Roth, E.C. Kleerup, S.H. Barsky, M.S. Simmons, and D.P. Tashkin. 1997. Tracheobronchial histopathology in habitual smokers of cocaine, marijuana and/or tobacco. *Chest* 112(2):319-326.

Frytak, S., C.G. Moertel, and J. Rubin. 1984. Metabolic studies of delta-9-tetrahydrocannabinol in cancer patients. *Cancer Treat Rep* 68(12):1427-1431.

Frytak, S., C.G. Moertel, J.R. O'Fallon, J. Rubin, E.T. Creagan, M.J. O'Connell, A.J. Schutt, and N.W. Schwartau. 1979. Delta-9-tetrahydrocannabinol as an antiemetic for patients receiving cancer chemotherapy. A comparison with prochlorperazine and a placebo. *Ann Intern Med* 91(6):825-830.

Gieringer, D. 1996. Marijuana research: Waterpipe study. *Bull Multidisc Assoc Psychedel Stud* 6(3):59-66.

Gieringer, D. 2000. Marijuana water pipe and vaporizer study. California NORML, San Francisco. http://www.maps.org/news-letters/v06n3/06359mj1.html

Gieringer, D. California NORML Press Release, January 7, 2001.

Gormeley, M. 2000. Associated Press. January 21.

Gorter, R., M. Seefried, and P. Volberding. 1992. Dronabinol effects on weight in patients with HIV infection. *AIDS* 6(1):127.

Guy G.W., and M.E. Flint. A phase one study of sublingual cannabis based medicinal extracts. 2000 Symposium on the Cannabinoids, Burlington, Vermont: International Cannabinoid Research Society, p. 115.

Hadgraft, J. 1996. Recent developments in topical and transdermal delivery. *Eur J Drug Metab Pharmacokinet* 21:165-173.

Hall, W., and N. Solowij. 1998. Adverse effects of cannabis. *Lancet* 352(9140): 1611-1616.

Hall, W., R. Room, and S. Bondy. 1999. Comparing the health and psychological risks of alcohol, cannabis nicotine and opiate use. In: H. Kalant, W. Corrigan, W. Hall, and R. Smart (eds.). *The health effects of cannabis.* Toronto: Addiction Research Foundation, pp. 477-508.

Holdcroft, A., M. Smith, A. Jacklin, H. Hodgson, B. Smith, M. Newton, and F. Evans. 1997. Pain relief with oral cannabinoids in familial Mediterranean fever. *Anaesthesia* 52(5):483-486.

Huber, G.L., and V.K. Mahajan. 1987. The comparative response of the lung to marihuana or tobacco smoke inhalation. In: Chesher, Greg, Paul Consroe, and Richard Musty. eds. *Marijuana: An international research report. Proceedings of Melbourne Symposium on Cannabis 2-4 September* (National Campaign Against Drug

Abuse Monograph Series No. 7, pp. 19-24). Canberra: Australian Government Publishing Service.

Jones, R.T., N.L. Benowitz, and R.I. Herning. 1981. Clinical relevance of cannabis tolerance and dependence. *J Clin Pharmacol* 21(8-9 Suppl):143S-152S.

Joy, J.E., S.J. Watson, Jr., and J.A. Benson, Jr. 1999. *Marijuana and medicine: Assessing the science base.* Institute of Medicine. Washington, DC: National Academy Press.

Lee, M.L., M. Novotny, and K.D. Bartle. 1976. Gas chromatography/mass spectrometric and nuclear magnetic resonance spectrometric studies of carcinogenic polynuclear aromatic hydrocarbons in tobacco and marijuana smoke condensates. *Anal Chem* 48(2):405-416.

Liguori, A., Gatto, C.P., and J.H. Robinson. 1998. Effects of marijuana on equilibrium, psychomotor performance, and simulated driving. *Behav Pharmacol* 9(7):590-609.

Lucas, V.S., Jr., and J. Laszlo. 1980. Δ9-tetrahydrocannabinol for refractory vomiting induced by cancer chemotherapy. *J Amer Med Assoc* 243(12):1241-1243.

Mattes, R.D., L.M. Shaw, and K. Engelman. 1994. Effects of cannabinoids (marijuana) on taste intensity and hedonic ratings and salivary flow of adults. *Chem Senses* 19(2):125-140.

McPartland, J.M. 2001. Contaminants and adulterants in herbal Cannabis. In: F. Grotenhermen, and E. Russo (eds.). *Cannabis and cannabinoids. Pharmacology, toxicology, and therapeutic potential.* Binghamton, NY: The Haworth Press, Inc., in press.

Meinck, H.M., P.W. Schönle, and B. Conrad. 1989. Effect of cannabinoids on spasticity and ataxia in multiple sclerosis. *J Neurol* 236(2):120-122.

Miller, W.E., R.E. Spiekerman, and N.G. Hepper. 1972. Pneumomediastinum resulting from performing Valsalva maneuvers during marihuana smoking. *Chest* 62(2): 233-234.

Mutschler E. 1996. *Arzneimittelwirkungen. Lehrbuch der Pharmakologie und Toxikologie.* 7th edition, Stuttgart: Wissenschaftliche Verlagsgesellschaft, p. 192.

Ohlsson, A., J.E. Lindgren, A. Wahlen, S. Agurell, L.E. Hollister, and H.K. Gillespie. 1980. Plasma delta-9 tetrahydrocannabinol concentrations and clinical effects after oral and intravenous administration and smoking. *Clin Pharmacol Ther* 28(3): 409-416.

O'Shaughnessy, W.B. 1838-1840. On the preparations of the Indian hemp or gunjah (*Cannabis indica*) Their effects on the animal system in health and their utility in the treatment of tetanus and other convulsive diseases. *Transactions of the Medical and Physical Society of Bengal* 1838-1840. Reprint in: Mikuriya, Tod H. ed. Marijuana: Medical Papers 1839-1972. Oakland: Medi-Comp Press, 1973.

Perez-Reyes, M., M.A. Lipton, M.C. Timmons, M.E. Wall, D.R. Brine, and K.H. Davis. 1973. Pharmacology of orally administered Δ9-tetrahydrocannabinol. *Clin Pharmacol Ther* 14(1):48-55.

Perez-Reyes, M., S.M. Owens, and S. Di Guiseppi. 1981. The clinical pharmacology and dynamics of marihuana cigarette smoking. *J Clin Pharmacol* 21(8-9 Suppl): 201S-207S.

Perlin, E., C.G. Smith, A.I. Nichols, R. Almirez, K.P. Flora, J.C. Cradock, and C.C. Peck. 1985. Disposition and bioavailability of various formulations of tetrahydrocannabinol in the rhesus monkey. *J Pharm Sci* 74(2):171-174.

Sherrill, D.L., M. Krzyzanowski, J.W. Bloom, and M.D. Lebowitz. 1991. Respiratory effects of non-tobacco cigarettes: A longitudinal study in general population. *Int J Epidemiol* 20(1):132-137.

Solowij, N., P.T. Michie, and A.M. Fox. 1991. Effects of long-term cannabis use on selective attention: An event-related potential study. *Pharmacol Biochem Behav* 40(3):683-688.

Sparacino, C.M., P.A. Hyldburg, and T.J. Hughes. 1990. Chemical and biological analysis of marijuana smoke condensate. *NIDA Res Monogr* 99:121-140.

Stevens, R.A., and S.M. Ghazi. 2000. Routes of opioid analgesic therapy in the management of cancer pain. *Cancer Control* 7(2):132-141.

Tashkin, D.P. 2001. Respiratory risks from marijuana smoking. In F. Grotenhermen, and E. Russo (eds.). *Cannabis and cannabinoids. Pharmacology, toxicology, and therapeutic potential.* Binghamton, NY: The Haworth Press, Inc., in press.

Tashkin, D.P., F. Gliederer, J. Rose, P. Chang, K.K. Hui, J.L. Yu, and T.C. Wu. 1991. Tar, CO and delta 9-THC delivery from the 1st and 2nd halves of a marijuana cigarette. *Pharmacol Biochem Behav* 40(3):657-661.

Tashkin, D.P., A.H. Coulson, V.A. Clark, M. Simmons, L.B. Bourque, S. Duann, G.H. Spivey, and H. Gong. 1987. Respiratory symptoms and lung function in habitual, heavy smokers of marijuana alone, smokers of marijuana and tobacco, smokers of tobacco alone, and nonsmokers. *Am Rev Resp Disease* 135:209-216.

Touitou, E., B. Fabin, S. Dany, and S. Almog. 1988. Transdermal delivery of tetrahydrocannabinol. *Int J Pharm* 43:9-15.

Touitou, E., and B. Fabin. 1988. Altered skin permeation of a highly lipophilic molecule: Tetrahydrocannabinol. *Int J Pharm* 43:17–22.

Turner, C.E., M.A. Elsohly, and E.G. Boeren. 1980. Constituents of *Cannabis sativa* L. XVII. A review of the natural constituents. *J Nat Prod* 43(2):169-234.

Ungerleider, J.T., T. Andrysiak, D.P. Tashkin, and R.P. Gale. 1982. Contamination of marihuana cigarettes with pathogenic bacteria-possible source of infection in cancer patients. *Cancer Treat Rep* 66(3):589-591.

Vaughan, C.W., and M.J. Christie. 2001. Mechanisms of cannabinoid analgesia. In F. Grotenhermen, and E. Russo (eds.). *Cannabis and cannabinoids. Pharmacology, toxicology, and therapeutic potential.* Binghamton, NY: The Haworth Press, Inc., in press.

Wall, M. E., B.M. Sadler, D. Brine, H. Taylor, and M. Perez-Reyes. 1983. Metabolism, disposition, and kinetics of delta-9-tetrahydrocannabinol in men and women. *Clin Pharmacol Ther* 34(3):352-363.

Wu, T.C., D.P. Tashkin, B. Djahed, and J.E. Rose. 1988. Pulmonary hazards of smoking marijuana as compared with tobacco. *N Engl J Med* 318(6):347-351.

Zhang, Z.-F., H. Morgenstern, M.R. Spitz, D.P. Tashkin, G.-P. Yu, J.R. Marshall, T.C. Hsu, S.P. Schantz. 1999. Marijuana use and increased risk of squamous cell carcinoma of the head and neck. *Cancer Epidemiol Biomarkers Prev* 8:1071-1079.

Cannabis "Vaporization":
A Promising Strategy
for Smoke Harm Reduction

Dale H. Gieringer

SUMMARY. The primary health hazard of medical cannabis is respiratory damage from marijuana smoke. Aside from oral ingestion and other non-smoked delivery systems not yet commercially available, strategies for reducing the harm of smoking include: (1) use of higher potency cannabis and (2) smoking devices aimed at eliminating toxins from the smoke. Studies have found that waterpipes and solid filters are ineffectual at improving the THC/tar ratio in cannabis smoke. The most promising alternative appears to be "vaporization," in which cannabis is heated to a point where cannabinoids are emitted without combustion. A feasibility study by NORML and MAPS has demonstrated that an electric vaporizer can successfully generate THC at 185°C while completely suppressing benzene, toluene, and naphthalene formation. Further studies are needed to evaluate how effectively vaporizers suppress other toxins, and how their performance varies using different samples, temperatures, and device designs. *[Article copies available for a fee from The Haworth Document Delivery Service: 1-800-342-9678. E-mail address: <getinfo@haworthpressinc.com> Website: <http://www.HaworthPress.com> © 2001 by The Haworth Press, Inc. All rights reserved.]*

Dale H. Gieringer, PhD, Coordinator, California NORML (National Organization for the Reform of Marijuana Laws) (E-mail: www.canorml.org; canorml@igc.org).

Address correspondence to: Dale H. Gieringer, PhD, 3514 Dwight Way, Berkeley, CA 94704.

The author thanks Rick Doblin, the Multidisciplinary Association for Psychedelic Studies, and Alternative Delivery Systems, Inc. for their indispensable support and assistance.

[Haworth co-indexing entry note]: "Cannabis 'Vaporization': A Promising Strategy for Smoke Harm Reduction." Gieringer, Dale H. Co-published simultaneously in *Journal of Cannabis Therapeutics* (The Haworth Integrative Healing Press, an imprint of The Haworth Press, Inc.) Vol. 1, No. 3/4, 2001, pp. 153-170; and: *Cannabis Therapeutics in HIV/AIDS* (ed: Ethan Russo) The Haworth Integrative Healing Press, an imprint of The Haworth Press, Inc., 2001, pp. 153-170. Single or multiple copies of this article are available for a fee from The Haworth Document Delivery Service [1-800-342-9678, 9:00 a.m. - 5:00 p.m. (EST). E-mail address: getinfo@haworthpressinc. com].

KEYWORDS. Marijuana, cannabis, smoke harm reduction, vaporizers, vaporization

INTRODUCTION

A leading health concern about the medical use of cannabis is respiratory sequelae due to smoking. Aside from its active cannabinoids, marijuana smoke greatly resembles tobacco smoke, containing noxious tars and gases that are a byproduct of leaf combustion. These include highly carcinogenic polycyclic aromatic hydrocarbons (PAHs) and other known carcinogens, such as benzene, at levels comparable to those in tobacco smoke. Also included are numerous other toxic inhalants, among them carbon monoxide, toluene, naphthalene, acetaldehyde, phenol, and hydrogen cyanide, again at levels comparable to tobacco (Huber 1991; Institute of Medicine 1982).

There is accordingly good reason to believe that chronic marijuana smoking poses many of the same respiratory hazards as tobacco. These hazards are offset by the fact that marijuana users typically consume a fraction as much material as tobacco smokers (1 g per day for a typical daily user, or 4 g per day for a very heavy, one-ounce per week medical patient, versus 20 g per day for a pack-a-day cigarette smoker). On the other hand, marijuana has been shown to deliver four times as much tar to the lungs per weight smoked as tobacco, possibly due to the deep breath holding of marijuana smokers (Wu et al. 1988).

On balance, the evidence indicates that marijuana smoking is not as great a public health hazard as tobacco. Epidemiological studies have yet to find evidence of lung cancer or increased mortality in frequent cannabis users (Sidney 1997a, 1997b). Unlike tobacco, cannabis lacks nicotine, a major risk factor in heart disease. Long-term studies of heavy users by Tashkin have found no evidence of a link between marijuana smoking and emphysema (Tashkin 1997, Zimmer and Morgan 1997).

Nonetheless, there is solid evidence to show a link between heavy cannabis smoking and respiratory disease. A succession of clinical studies have found that long-term, frequent marijuana smokers exhibit signs of respiratory damage, including chronic bronchitis, sore throat, inflammation, impaired immune function, and pre-cancerous cell changes (Tashkin 1993). A survey of patients at the Kaiser Permanente medical centers found that marijuana smokers suffered a significantly higher incidence of respiratory complaints (Polen et al. 1993). There have also been anecdotal reports of neck and throat cancers in heavy marijuana smokers, most of whom also smoked tobacco. Another concern in light of the widespread use of cannabis among AIDS patients is that heavy marijuana smoking might increase susceptibility to lung infections such as *Pneumocystis carinii* pneumonia, although such a risk has not been proven.

In sum, respiratory harm has been rightly called "the only well-confirmed deleterious physical effect of marijuana" in the words of Dr. Lester Grinspoon (Grinspoon 1997, p. 250). Given the growing public pressure against smoking tobacco, these concerns have loomed large as an obstacle to acceptance of medical marijuana by public health authorities. In its review of medical marijuana, the Institute of Medicine of the National Academy of Sciences found "no future" in smoked marijuana, saying, "Because marijuana is a crude delivery system that also delivers harmful substances, smoked marijuana should generally not be recommended for medical use" (Institute of Medicine 1999, pp. 10-11). However, the IOM failed to consider various harm reduction techniques that might substantially reduce the hazards associated with smoking cannabis.

In this study, we will discuss the state of the art of marijuana smoke harm reduction, focusing particularly on smoking devices such as waterpipes and vaporizers aimed at reducing the toxins in cannabis smoke. Before doing so, however, it is worth briefly discussing other strategies for respiratory harm reduction.

SMOKE HARM REDUCTION STRATEGIES

The most obvious alternative to marijuana smoking is to ingest cannabis orally via tinctures, extracts, foodstuffs, or capsules. The limitations of oral dosages are well known and substantial (Grinspoon 1997). Oral THC is notoriously unreliable in its effects. The bioavailability of oral cannabinoids varies greatly depending on the individual patient and the state of his or her metabolism and digestive system. Unlike inhaled cannabis, the effects of which become readily apparent within seconds, allowing the patient to regulate the dose via self-titration, oral dosages require up to an hour or more to take effect. Over- or under-dosage is therefore a common problem. The delayed onset of oral cannabis also renders it unsuitable for conditions requiring prompt treatment, such as acute pain or convulsions. In addition, oral dosages are hard to keep down for patients suffering intense nausea. Finally, oral dosages do not have the same pharmacological action as inhaled marijuana, since orally ingested THC does not pass directly into the bloodstream, as with smoking, but is rather processed by the liver, where it is transformed into another, even more psychoactive metabolite, 11-hydroxy-THC (Zimmer and Morgan 1997). The medical implications of this are unknown, though they might include an increased risk of adverse "panic reactions." Historically, the declining interest in medical cannabis at the turn of the last century was attributed to the unreliability of its effects, which may be explained by its oral dosage form. The manifold drawbacks of oral preparations such as synthetic oral THC (dronabinol,

's patients to prefer inhaled marijuana; how-
s patients found only minor differences in the
oked herbal cannabis (Corral 2001).
dministration have been proposed, but have
ial fruition. Topical applications such as can-
ed in folk medicine, but their efficacy is dubi-
transdermal cannabinoid patch was recently
General Hydroponics (US Patent 6,113,940;
ml), but its efficacy has yet to be demon-
is not suited for transdermal application be-
Institute of Medicine 1999), the possibility
ally active cannabis derivatives can be trans-

een proposed to treat glaucoma, but have yet
SA (Grinspoon 1997; Green et al. 1976).
system has been demonstrated by ElSohly us-
o-drug that transforms into THC. This could
dronabinol for patients with extreme nausea.
ensed development by Oxford Natural Prod-

ve to smoked marijuana would seem to be
r. Attempts to aerosolize THC have encoun-
past (Tashkin 1977). However, Pertwee has
ment of a cannabis spray based on a new, wa-
leveloped in collaboration with Razdan and
xpected within five or ten years (BBC News
very systems for synthetic THC (dronabinol,
d in Phase I studies by Unimed: deep lung
d sublingual preparations (Institute of Medi-
ms for natural cannabis extracts are under in-
als in the U.K. (Hadorn 2001). New delivery
for marketing in the next few years, at least
ir usage and availability will be limited by li-
s to certain approved products. For the fore-
erefore continue to find them unobtainable or

oked marijuana is therefore likely to remain
orm of cannabis, both medicinally and other-
to how to reduce its harmfulness to the respi-

igher-potency sinsemilla (Spanish for "with-
o as to boost the proportion of THC in the

(HIV-1MN). (
tionally to car
The CB_1-selec
tion of the int
nonselective
versed the SR
antagonist cou
intracellular p.

Because in
a complex net
upon exposure
may lead to ad
terized by aug
Massi et al. (2
volved in med
by THC was p
though the CI
strated, also, th
of IFNγ produ
who indicated
IL-12, and IL-
Furthermore,
were attenuate
of the Th1-pro
Coy et al. (19
comes may be
observed that
macrophage p
of hen egg lys
fects by both r
type. Felder e
receptor- and r
cell lines whic
expression vec
their studies.
CP55940 indi
cAMP accum
ceptor-linked
arachidonic ac
functional link
Whether ca
non-receptor r

smoke, thereby necessitating a smaller intake of smoke. Obviously, this assumes that patients can reliably adjust their smoke intake to deliver a given desired dose of cannabinoids. It also assumes that the smoke from higher-potency preparations delivers proportionately higher ratios of cannabinoids to toxins–an assumption that may not hold if their chemical consistency and combustion properties are substantially different from that of regular cannabis.

SMOKING DEVICES

Another promising strategy for smoke harm reduction is to separate or eliminate the harmful toxins from the useful cannabinoids via some sort of purification or filtration device. A profusion of smoking devices are currently available on the underground market and are in use by medical marijuana patients. Although most have no evident health benefits, a few purport to offer harm reduction attributes.

Assuming that patients aim to achieve a given dose of cannabinoids, the proper measure for smoke harm reduction should be the overall ratio of cannabinoids to toxins. The higher this ratio, the fewer the noxious smoke byproducts patients have to take into their lungs in order to achieve a given effective dose.

Three basic kinds of smoking devices are presently in use for marijuana smoke harm reduction:

- *Waterpipes:* Marijuana smoke can be inhaled through waterpipes, bongs or similar devices in the hopes of cleansing the smoke via water filtration. Many patients strongly prefer to smoke cannabis through waterpipes, feeling that they deliver smoother, cooler, less irritating smoke. Studies indicate that water filtration can be effective in reducing tars and other toxins in tobacco and marijuana smoke (Cozzi 1993). The problem is that such devices may also filter out medically active cannabinoids, degrading the actual cannabinoid/toxin ratio (Gieringer 1996).
- *Solid filters:* Smoke can also be inhaled through solid filters such as those in tobacco cigarettes. Cigarette filters are known to produce modest reductions in tobacco smoke tars, and can also be used with cannabis. Once again, the problem is that they also filter out active THC (Gieringer 1996). The essential question therefore remains as to whether solid filters can actually improve the cannabinoid/toxin ratio.
- *Vaporizers:* Observations by users and laboratory studies described below indicate that it is possible to generate psychoactive vapors from cannabis by heating it to a temperature below the point of combustion, where the bulk of carcinogens are formed. This process is popularly re-

ferred to as "vaporization" or "volatilization." (In actuality, the exact physical process is uncertain: the Merck Index lists the vaporization point of THC as 200°C *in vacuo*, but users have reported psychoactive vapors at temperatures ≤180°C under normal atmospheric pressure.) In theory, an ideal vaporizer would deliver a stream of medically active cannabinoids without any of the toxic byproducts of combustion. In practice, experimental vaporizers are observed to produce a light stream of apparently cannabinoid-laced vapors, without heavy smoke or ash, leaving the marijuana crisped with a toasted, green-to greenish-brown appearance. Although numerous models of vaporizers are currently available on the market, none have been subjected to FDA-style efficacy testing, and they remain technically illegal for medical cannabis use under current paraphernalia laws.

Until recently, there has been little scientific basis on which to judge the alternative marijuana smoking harm reduction strategies. However, a handful of recent studies have begun to shed light on the subject.

NORML/MAPS SMOKING DEVICE STUDY

In an effort to evaluate the feasibility of marijuana smoking harm reduction, California NORML (National Organization for the Reform of Marijuana Laws) and MAPS (Multidisciplinary Association for Psychedelic Studies) sponsored a study of seven different smoking devices: three different water-pipes, two electric vaporizers, a joint fitted with a cigarette filter, plus a regular unfiltered joint as a control (Gieringer 1996). The study was designed to assess the ratio of cannabinoids to tar for each device, on the theory that higher THC/tar ratios would correlate with reduced respiratory hazards.

Samples of government-supplied marijuana from the National Institute on Drug Abuse (NIDA) were puffed in a smoking machine in a manner designed to mimic human marijuana smoking. The smoke was collected in Cambridge glass fiber filters designed to capture particles > 0.1 microns, which are used to separate solid particulates or "tars" from gaseous smoke components such as carbon monoxide. The filtered solids also include all of the cannabinoids. The filtered residue was weighed to measure total tar content and quantitatively analyzed for three cannabinoids, THC, CBD and CBN, by means of a gas chromatograph/mass spectrometer (GC/MS).

As expected, all of the devices produced a reduction in tars relative to the control: 33% for the filter, 89%-98% for the waterpipes, and 56%-97% for the vaporizers (Table 1). However, only the vaporizers achieved an improvement in the ratio of tars to cannabinoids. The cigarette filter performed worse than

TABLE 1. Tar and Cannabinoid Delivery–7 Smoking Devices

	Nonfilter Cigarette	Filter Cigarette	Waterpipe #1	Waterpipe #2	Waterpipe #3	Vaporizer #1	Vaporizer #2
Total Tars (mg/puff)	309.8	140.5	24.5	9.2	78.3	4.76	11.3
Total Cannabinoids (% Tar)	7.82	5.32	5.46	4.48	2.50	7.89	9.82
Total THC (%Tar)	5.99	4.12	4.31	2.14	3.36	6.27	5.24

Adapted from Gieringer, D. "Marijuana Waterpipe and Vaporizer Study," 1996

the unfiltered joint, producing 30% more tar per cannabinoids. Worse yet were the waterpipes, which produced from 30% to 180% more tars per cannabinoids. Ironically, the worst waterpipes were those designed to maximize the vapor's exposure to water. The disappointing implication is that waterpipes may actually be counterproductive in reducing tars from cannabis smoking.

A likely explanation for the poor performance of physical filtration systems is that THC molecules are especially sticky and apt to adhere to other smoke particles. Any attempt to screen out the latter is therefore apt to pick up the former as well. Indeed, to the extent that cannabinoids are relatively stickier than other compounds, particles containing them may be more likely to be trapped by filters.

The vaporizers were the only devices to outperform the unfiltered joint, though only by a modest margin. The first vaporizer, a commercial model consisting of a battery-powered metal hot plate inside a jar to trap the vapor, achieved a 26% improvement in the cannabinoid/tar ratio. The second model, a homemade, hybrid device, consisting of a hot air gun blowing through a beaker of water, combined vaporization with water filtration. It achieved a statistically insignificant 0.25% improvement. However, its performance may well have been degraded by the water filtration component, the inclusion of which seemed in retrospect to be a design flaw in the experiment.

Evaluation of the vaporizers was further complicated by the fact that the "hot plate" model produced anomalously high amounts of CBN and 30% less THC. The origins of the CBN are not certain, but might well be due to partial pyrolysis of THC (Fehr and Kalant 1972). Since CBN has negligible pharmacological activity compared to THC, it seemed appropriate to recompute the device performances in terms of the ratio of THC to tars. When this was done, the hotplate turned out to be 13% worse than the unfiltered joint, while the hot air device was 4.6% better.

The most disappointing finding of the smoking device study was the apparent counter-productivity of waterpipes and cigarette filters. However, this conclusion must be qualified by several important caveats due to limitations in the study design:

- The gaseous component of the smoke was not analyzed in the study. Cannabis smoke contains numerous noxious gases, including hydrogen cyanide, which incapacitates the lung's defensive cilia, volatile phenols, which contribute to the harshness of the taste, aldehydes, which promote cancer, and carbon monoxide, a known risk factor in heart disease (Huber 1991). There is evidence that water filtration may be quite effective in absorbing some of these gases, especially those that are water-soluble (Cozzi 1993). If so, waterpipes could still turn out to have some health benefits.
- The study did not attempt to quantify the specific chemical components of the tars except for the cannabinoids. It is conceivable that the tars from the waterpipe or cigarette filter contained relatively less harmful toxins and carcinogens, and more inert ingredients, than the unfiltered ones.
- In conformity with cigarette smoking conventions, a 30-cm butt length was left unsmoked on the unfiltered joint. Thus, the study did not test the last part of the joint, the "roach," which is commonly savored to complete exhaustion by marijuana connoisseurs. The roach is known to accumulate higher concentrations of tars and THC from the rest of the cigarette (Tashkin et al. 1991a). It is possible that the cannabinoid/tar ratio for the unfiltered joint would have been considerably different if the roach had been included. It is also possible that there are other ways in which the smoking machine did not accurately replicate the inhalation pattern of human smokers.

Although the vaporizers showed at best marginal effectiveness in the study, substantial improvements might have been realized with more careful research and development. Neither vaporizer was carefully designed, adjusted, or optimized for laboratory testing. Furthermore, unlike waterpipes and filtration devices, vaporizers are at least based on a physical principle that offers a theoretical hope for further development. For this reason, NORML and MAPS decided to undertake a second study devoted specifically to vaporizers, preliminary results of which are presented below.

SOUTH AUSTRALIAN GOVERNMENT STUDY

A study sponsored by the South Australian Drug and Alcohol Services Council confirmed the apparent inefficacy of waterpipes, while raising confusing new issues about marijuana smoke harm reduction (Gowing et al. 2000).

The study tested 12 different varieties of cannabis, ranging from low-grade leaf to high-potency sinsemilla. All samples were dried, trimmed, shredded and homogenized in a blender. The samples were smoked in standard joints, in waterpipes, and in combination with tobacco using a Filtrona smoking machine under standard cigarette smoking conditions. Particulate matter was trapped in Cambridge type glass fiber filters. The smoke was analyzed for THC yield, tar, water, and carbon monoxide.

The study found that the waterpipes consistently generated more tars and carbon monoxide than the unfiltered cigarettes. Tar yields were on the order of 3 to 7 times higher per given sample, while carbon monoxide was 2 to 4 times higher. Unfortunately, no comparative data on THC yield were produced, making it impossible to assess the overall THC/tar and CO ratios. Nonetheless, the researchers concluded that the risks of cannabis smoking were less likely to be reduced by a waterpipe as opposed to a cigarette.

A significant part of the difference between waterpipes and cigarettes could be explained by differences in smoking conditions. Whereas the cigarettes had been puffed at 60-second intervals, the waterpipes had to be puffed at 6-second intervals in order to keep them lit. When the cigarettes were re-tested at 6-second intervals, it was found that two-thirds of the increase in tar content and one-third of the increase in CO were accounted for. (Again, there were no THC data to assess what change may have occurred in the relative THC/tar and CO ratios.) Another factor that could have explained the higher tar from the waterpipe was that the cigarettes were smoked to a butt length of 23 mm, while the waterpipe smoke was drawn directly into the smoking machine. Hence, the butt may have filtered out more tars and CO from the cigarette smoke.

A startling finding of the study was that the composition of the smoke varied widely depending on the specific samples and smoking conditions. In particular, THC yields varied radically for different samples and devices. In the case of cigarettes, no clear correlation was observed between the potency of cannabis smoked and the amount of THC actually delivered in the smoke. One cigarette of 0.69% THC leaf delivered smoke of 0.62% THC content, while another cigarette of 12.97% flowering "heads" yielded only 0.54% THC in smoke, a remarkable 25-fold difference in efficiency of THC delivery. In the case of waterpipes, smoke and sample potency were better correlated, although not in full proportion. For example, high-grade samples of 9-13% potency yielded no more than 2.4% THC in waterpipe smoke, while low-grade samples of 2% yielded amounts ranging from 0.08% to 1.1%. These results are strikingly at variance with the observations of many experienced users, who report that one or two tokes (inhalations) of good, high-grade sinsemilla can be equivalent to a whole cigarette of regular cannabis. Such discrepancies may be explained by peculiarities in the particular samples tested or by systematic differences between human smoking and the laboratory smoking machine used in the Australian study. In any event, the Australian study implies that higher cannabis potency does not necessarily translate to more available THC.

The investigators inferred that actual THC delivery is highly dependent on the particular sample and smoking conditions, including puff length, temperature, and other factors. In particular, tests showed a significant, positive correlation between THC delivery and water content of the smoke for both cigarettes and waterpipes. It is unknown how the water content of the smoke was related to the original water content of the samples as opposed to other factors, such as temperature of combustion. For example, it is possible that excessively moist samples could have produced *less* water and THC in the smoke if they burned less efficiently. The most that can be concluded is that THC yield is related to factors that are also related to water yield. It has been proposed that THC is normally released not via pyrolysis or volatilization, but by a process of co-distillation with steam, in which cannabinoids are expelled along with water vapor in the 2 mm high temperature gradient zone before the burning front (Fehr and Kalant 1972). This hypothesis seems bolstered by the finding that THC and water yield are correlated.

Further evidence for the importance of smoking conditions with respect to THC yield was seen when tobacco was added to the cannabis. When mixed with 50% tobacco and 50% cannabis, the cigarettes yielded between 93% less and 81% *more* THC. The waterpipes performed more consistently with expectations, yielding 30-55% less THC in most cases. Tar levels increased when tobacco was added to cigarettes but generally held steady for waterpipes, while carbon monoxide increased for both, though more so in waterpipes. The samples that had the worst THC delivery in cigarettes showed the most marked improvement when combined with tobacco. This suggested that the tobacco had made the samples burn better, perhaps by raising the temperature so as to release more THC.

VAPORIZER STUDIES

The theory supporting vaporization has been known for sometime. A vaporizer known as the Tilt was commercially marketed in the early 1980's before passage of the anti-paraphernalia laws. Its performance was investigated in an unpublished study for the manufacturer by a graduate research assistant at MIT (Herms 1978). Although the Tilt is no longer available, the study report provides good evidence for the feasibility of vaporization.

The Tilt consisted of a wire sample screen mounted 5 mm above an adjustable 80-watt radiant heater, all encased in a plastic chamber with an exit port near the top (Diagram 1). In the study, samples of unpowdered cannabis buds and fragments were placed on the screen and held at constant temperatures

DIAGRAM 1. Tilt Advertisement

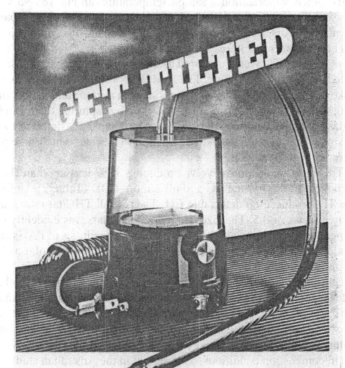

Now you can reduce the hazards of smoking. Without reducing the pleasures. With The Tilt, the world's most intelligently engineered smoking system.

Instead of burning your smoking materials, The Tilt heats them electronically. Just enough to release their active ingredients... at their height of potency.

There's no combustion, so there's up to 96%* less tar in your smoke. Less bite and harshness. Nothing comes through but the richest essences of your smoking materials. And more of them, because ingredients destroyed by burning are released intact by The Tilt.

So if you don't plan to quit smoking, take up Tilting... the intelligent alternative.

Order The Tilt with a toll-free call (credit cards only) or the coupon below.

THE TILT.
THE ULTIMATE SMOKING SYSTEM.

while the vapors were drawn off by suction. The lab reported that the Tilt achieved efficient vaporization at sample temperatures around 185-95°C. This is similar to the temperature range used by patients today. The sample exuded a thin stream of vapors, but kept its green color. Spontaneous combustion was reported at sample temperatures above 200°C.

Vapors from the Tilt were compared to smoke produced by similar samples combusted in a common clay pipe. THC and CBD were measured by capturing the smoke in a cold trap, dissolving the residues in acetone and methanol, and analyzing them via GC/MS. Tars were measured by capturing them in a Cambridge glass filter and weighing them. Carbon monoxide was detected by passing the smoke through a solution of palladium chloride, which precipitates palladium in the presence of CO.

The Tilt performed impressively, producing 79% less tar than the pipe while producing 80% more THC and 60% more CBD (Table 2). Unlike the pipe, the Tilt produced no detectable CO. The overall THC/tar ratio was improved by a factor of 8.5. The sizeable reduction in tars was evidently due to the absence of combustion, which forms hazardous quantities of PAHs at temperatures above 560-600°C (Wynder and Hoffmann 1967). Insofar as PAHs are thought to constitute the major carcinogenic hazard of smoking, the Tilt would seem to have offered substantial harm reduction benefits. Another remarkable feat of the Tilt was to generate more available cannabinoids than the pipe. The report speculated that this was because cannabinoids undergo degradative reactions such as polymerization, cyclization, etc., at combustion temperatures of 600° or more. However, a more likely explanation may be differences in combustion conditions, as observed in the Australian study.

NORML/MAPS VAPORIZATION STUDY

In order to further explore the potential of vaporization, California NORML and MAPS have undertaken a second, new vaporizer research project. The project is focusing on two models of vaporizers that are currently available and

TABLE 2. Pipe Smoke Compared to Vapor from Tilt Vaporizer

	Smoke from clay pipe	Vapor from Tilt
Delta-9-THC	0.044%	0.079%
Cannabidiol	0.015%	0.024%
"Tar"	16.5%	3.4%
Carbon Monoxide	Present	Absent

Adapted from Herms 1978

in use by medical marijuana patients: an electric radiator similar to the Tilt, and a hot air gun. The first phase of the project, a preliminary "proof of concept" study of the first device, is now complete. The results confirm that cannabinoid vapors can be generated around 185°C with substantial reductions in certain smoke toxins. Further studies are currently in progress.

The preliminary study tested a device called the M1 Volatizer (Figure 1), an aromatherapy device developed by Alternative Delivery Systems, Inc., consisting of an electric heating element arranged to radiate heat over a sample placed on a wire screen in a standard glass bong bowl. The sample consisted of sifted, cured sinsemilla cannabis (Figure 2). Temperature was regulated by a rheostat and measured via a themocoupled electronic thermometer on the sample. Vapors were drawn off with a vacuum pump and analyzed in three separate tests for: (1) carbon monoxide, (2) particulate matter, and (3) six target analyses: three cannabinoids (THC, CBD and CBN), and three toxic aromatic hydrocarbons, benzene, a known carcinogen, plus toluene and naphthalene.

Results showed that the vaporizer produced qualitative reduction in CO and particulates and complete elimination of the three toxic hydrocarbons (Table 3).

- Carbon monoxide was tested semi-quantitatively by drawing the sample for 20 seconds through a Drager tube. The M1 was operated at the comparatively low sample temperature of 170°C, where it produced a light gray vapor. Unlike the Tilt, the M1 produced detectable carbon monoxide (although the sensitivity of the Tilt CO test is unknown). When combusted with a match, the sample produced a thick, dark gray smoke. Unfortunately, the combustion test saturated the Drager tube, making it impossible to quantify the change in CO. The most that could be determined was that the M1 reduced CO by ≥33% compared to combustion.
- Particulate matter was measured by passing the smoke through a Balston Microfibre Disposable Filter Unit. The M1 was maintained at 185°C for 3 min and 45 secs and the vacuum pump run simultaneously for 5 min. A second sample was combusted with a match and the vacuum pump run for 5 min. The filter from the M1 showed slight discoloration at the top, while the filter from the combusted sample was saturated with yellow discoloration. The net particulate weight in the filter was at least 56% less using the vaporizer. Once again, however, it was impossible to measure the full extent of the reduction, since the combusted smoke appeared to have completely saturated the second filter.
- The three cannabinoids and three toxic hydrocarbons were measured by passing the vapors through a methanol-filled collection flask. The M1 was held at 185°C for three minutes and the vacuum pump run for 5 minutes. The control sample was combusted with a match with the vacuum pump running for three minutes. The contents of the flask were removed

and assayed using a High Performance Liquid Chromatograph-Diode Array Detector-Mass Spectrometer. The three toxic hydrocarbons (benzene, toluene and naphthalene) were all detected in the combusted smoke, but not in the vaporized output. Unlike the Tilt, the M1 produced 85% less THC than combustion. There were indications that THC production could have been improved by refinements in laboratory technique. In any event, there was a 100% reduction in the toxin/THC ratio.

Data were insufficient to evaluate changes in CBD and CBN. (Users of the M1 have reported that they obtain different psychoactive effects at different temperatures, suggesting possible variations in the proportions of different cannabinoids.)

IMPLICATIONS FOR RESPIRATORY HARM REDUCTION

Results so far are tentative and incomplete, but promising. Clearly, much work needs to be done to explore the effects of different adjustments and smoking conditions. NORML and MAPS are currently sponsoring more research to determine how temperature affects the production of THC and other cannabinoids relative to other toxins. Tests indicate that small amounts of THC may be released at temperatures as low as 140°C. Significant amounts of

FIGURE 1. M1 Volatizer

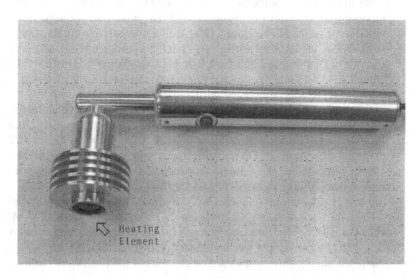

TABLE 3. M1 Vaporizer Performance: Reduction in Presence of Compounds Under Vaporization at 185°C Relative to Combustion

	Particulate "Tar"	Benzene	Toluene	Naphthalene	Carbon Monoxide*	THC
Reduction	> 56%	100%	100%	100%	> 33%	85%

*CO vaporization temperature 170°

FIGURE 2. Effect of Vaporization

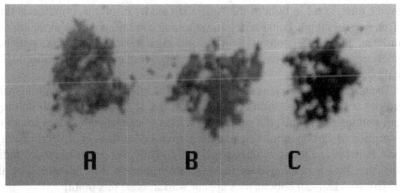

A = Crude sinsemilla (olive green)
B = Similar specimen after vaporization by hot air gun at 180°C for ~5 min (brownish green)
C = Similar specimen after combustion (black)

benzene, toluene and naphthalene were observed above 200°C, and combustion occurred at temperatures of 230°C or higher. Further work is necessary to ascertain how these temperatures vary for samples of different humidity, potency, composition, and consistency. It is reasonable to assume that the vaporizer can completely avoid production of the highly carcinogenic PAHs, since these require pyrolysis to form. There is accordingly good reason to think that vaporizers can substantially reduce the presence of carcinogens in marijuana smoke. The question of carbon monoxide and other toxins is more uncertain. NORML and MAPS are seeking to explore these issues in future research. From the Australian work, it also seems likely that the performance of vaporizers and other smoking devices is critically dependent on the particular cannabis sample, its preparation and curing, variations in smoking technique, and other factors. These issues remain to be researched. In the meantime, vaporizers are becoming increasingly popular with medical cannabis patients, who report they are far less irritating than other methods of smoking.

Aside from vaporization, the one remaining strategy for cannabis smoke harm reduction is to use stronger THC preparations. Studies to date have found little evidence that users self-titrate dosage according to the potency of cannabis being smoked (Chait 1989; Zimmer and Morgan 1997). However, research has been restricted to a limited, low potency range (typically 0%-3%), using standard NIDA-issued leaf cigarettes. To date, no studies have been done with the kind of high-grade sinsemilla now widely available to patients through medical cannabis clubs, the potency of which may range from 8% to 20% or greater (Gieringer 1996). Lack of research in this area remains a grievous deficiency. The usefulness of high-grade sinsemilla for smoke harm reduction may be questioned in light of the Australian study, insofar as it indicates that differences in sample consistency and smoking conditions can be more important than the THC content of marijuana cigarettes. Nonetheless, patients widely report that they can effectively reduce smoke inhalation using high-quality sinsemilla.

The hazards of marijuana smoke may also be affected by the breathing pattern of the user. Some studies have suggested that prolonged breath holding does nothing to enhance the subjective effects of cannabis, but does increase absorption of carbon monoxide and other toxins (Azorlosa et al. 1995; Zacny and Chait 1991; Zimmer and Morgan 1997). However, other evidence indicates that breath holding does increase absorption of THC (Tashkin et al. 1991b). No clear-cut conclusions appear warranted at this point.

There is an evident need for further research on cannabis vaporization and marijuana smoke harm reduction. Sadly, due to the political fallout of the war on drugs, the government or leading private health research foundations are not supporting such research.

REFERENCES

Azorlosa, J., M. Greenwald and M. Stitzer. 1995. Marijuana smoking: effects of varying puff volume and breathhold duration. *J Pharmacol Exper Therap* 272: 560-9.

BBC News. 2000. Scientists develop cannabis spray. (UK Web) BBC Feedback: 11 December.

Chait, L.D. 1989. Delta-9-tetrahydrocannabinol content and human marijuana self-administration. *Psychopharmacol* 98: 51-5.

Corral, V. 2001. Differential effects of medical marijuana based on strain and route of administration: a three-year observational study. *J Cannabis Therap* 1(3/4):43-59.

Cozzi, N. 1993. Effects of water filtration on marijuana smoke: a literature review. *MAPS Bull* 4(2):4-6.

ElSohly, M. 2000. Personal communication 11 December.

Fehr, K.O. and H. Kalant. 1972. Analysis of cannabis smoke obtained under different combustion conditions. *Canad J Physiol Pharmacol* 50:761-7.

Gieringer, D. 1996. Marijuana waterpipe and vaporizer study, *MAPS Bull* 6(3):59-66. Multidisciplinary Association for Psychedelic Studies, www.maps.org/news-letters/v06n3/06359mj1.html

Gieringer, D. 1999. Medical cannabis potency testing project, *MAPS Bull* 9(3):20-2. Multidisciplinary Association for Psychedelic Studies, www.maps.org/news-letters/v09n3/09320gie.html

Gowing, L., R. Ali and J. White. 2000. Respiratory harms of smoked cannabis, Research Monograph No. 8. Adelaide: Drug and Alcohol Services Council of South Australia.

Green, K., K. Kim and K. Bowman. 1976. Ocular effects of delta-9-tetrahydrocannabinol, in S. Cohen and R. Stillman (eds.). *The therapeutic potential of marihuana*. New York and London: Plenum Medical Book Co. pp. 49-62.

Grinspoon, L. 1997. *Marijuana, the forbidden medicine*. Revised edition. New Haven: Yale University Press.

Hadorn, D. 2001. Personal communication (North American Medical Director, GW Pharmaceuticals).

Herms, J. 1978. Letter to Mr. Robert Tabatznik of RTA Inc., Woodstock, NY. MIT Department of Material Science. Dated 3 December.

Huber, G., M. First and O. Grubner. 1991. Marijuana and tobacco smoke gas-phase cytotoxins. *Pharmacol Biochem Behav* 40:629-36.

Institute of Medicine. 1982. *Marijuana and health*. Washington, DC: National Academy Press.

Institute of Medicine. 1999. *Marijuana and medicine: Assessing the science base*. Washington, DC: National Academy Press.

Polen, M., S. Sidney, I. Tekawa, M. Sadler and G. Friedman. 1993. Health care use by frequent marijuana smokers who do not smoke tobacco. *West J Med* 158:596-601.

Sidney, S., J. Beck, I. Tekawa, C. Quisenberry and G. Friedman. 1997a. Marijuana use and mortality. *Amer J Publ Health* 87:585-90.

Sidney, S., C. Quisenberry, G. Friedman and I. Tekawa. 1997b. Marijuana use and cancer incidence (California, United States). *Cancer Cause and Control* 8: 722-8.

Tashkin, D., S. Reiss, B. Shapiro, B. Calvarese, J. Olsen and J. Lodge 1977. Bronchial effects of aerosolized delta-9-tetrahydrocannabinol in healthy and asthmatic subjects. *Amer Rev Resp Dis* 115:57-65.

Tashkin, D., F. Gliederer, J. Rose, P. Chang, K.K. Hui, J.L. Yu and T-C. Wu. 1991a. Tar, CO and delta-9 THC delivery from the 1st and 2nd halves of a marijuana cigarette. *Pharmacol Bioch Behav* 40:657-61.

Tashkin, D., F. Gliederer, J. Rose, P. Chang, K.K. Hui, J.L. Yu and T-C. Wu. 1991b. Effects of varying marijuana smoking profile on deposition of tar and absorption of CO and delta-9-THC. *Pharmacol Biochem Behav* 40:651-6.

Tashkin, D. 1993. Is frequent marijuana smoking harmful to health? *West J Med* 158:635-7.

Tashkin, D. 1997. Heavy habitual marijuana smoking does not cause an accelerated decline in FEV_1 with age. *Amer J Resp Crit Care Med* 155:141-8.

Wu, T-C., D. Tashkin, B. Djahed and J. Rose 1988. Pulmonary hazards of smoking marijuana as compared with tobacco. *New Engl J Med* 318:347-51.

Wynder, E. and D. Hoffman. 1967. *Tobacco and tobacco smoke*. New York: Academic Press, pp. 346-9.

Zacny, J. and L. Chait. 1991. Response to marijuana as a function of potency and breathhold duration. *Psychopharmacol* 103:223-6.

Zimmer, L. and J. Morgan. 1997. *Marijuana myths, marijuana facts: A review of the scientific evidence*. New York and San Francisco: Lindesmith Center.

Analgesic and Reinforcing Properties of Δ9-THC-Hemisuccinate in Adjuvant-Arthritic Rats

Susan L. Broom
Kenneth J. Sufka
Mahmoud A. ElSohly
Samir A. Ross

SUMMARY. The use of Δ9-THC hemisuccinate (HS) in a suppository formulation is an attempt to develop a cannabinoid possessing possible therapeutic effects with a minimal side effect profile. The purpose of this study was to investigate the antinociceptive and reinforcing effects of rectally administered Δ9-THC-HS in rats. Tests were conducted in two groups of animals: Complete Freund's adjuvant-inflamed animals (CFA)

Susan L. Broom, MA, is Psychology Graduate Research Assistant, University of Mississippi, University, MS 38677.

Kenneth J. Sufka, PhD, is Associate Professor of Psychology and Pharmacology, University of Mississippi, University, MS 38677.

Mahmoud A. ElSohly, PhD, is Professor of Pharmaceutics, Research Professor, National Center for Natural Products Research, University of Mississippi, University, MS 38677, and is President, ElSohly Laboratories, Oxford, MS 38655.

Samir A. Ross, PhD, is Associate Professor of Pharmacognosy, Associate Research Professor, National Center for Natural Products Research, University of Mississippi, University, MS 38677.

Address correspondence to: Kenneth J. Sufka, PhD, Associate Professor of Psychology and Pharmacology, Peabody Building, University of Mississippi, University, MS 38677 (E-mail: pysufka@olemiss.edu).

[Haworth co-indexing entry note]: "Analgesic and Reinforcing Properties of Δ9-THC-Hemisuccinate in Adjuvant-Arthritic Rats." Broom, Susan L. et al. Co-published simultaneously in *Journal of Cannabis Therapeutics* (The Haworth Integrative Healing Press, an imprint of The Haworth Press, Inc.) Vol. 1, No. 3/4, 2001, pp. 171-182; and: *Cannabis Therapeutics in HIV/AIDS* (ed: Ethan Russo) The Haworth Integrative Healing Press, an imprint of The Haworth Press, Inc., 2001, pp. 171-182. Single or multiple copies of this article are available for a fee from The Haworth Document Delivery Service [1-800-342-9678, 9:00 a.m. - 5:00 p.m. (EST). E-mail address: getinfo@haworthpressinc.com].

and non-inflamed controls. A hotplate test was administered to index hyperalgesia and possible analgesic effects of Δ^9-THC-HS on thermal nociception. CFA animals demonstrated shorter latencies than non-inflamed animals. The highest dose of Δ^9-THC-HS produced longer hotplate latencies. Additionally, the reinforcing properties of Δ^9-THC-HS were evaluated using the Conditioned Place Preference (CPP) paradigm. Δ^9-THC-HS produced an increase in preference scores in non-inflamed animals (positive reinforcement), but did not affect preference scores in CFA animals. These data suggest that Δ^9-THC-HS has therapeutic potential and is unlikely to possess an abuse liability when used in the context of chronic pain. *[Article copies available for a fee from The Haworth Document Delivery Service: 1-800-342-9678. E-mail address: <getinfo@ haworthpressinc.com> Website: <http://www.HaworthPress.com> © 2001 by The Haworth Press, Inc. All rights reserved.]*

KEYWORDS. Δ^9-THC, adjuvant-inflamed, rat, hotplate, conditioned place preference

INTRODUCTION

The role of cannabinoids (CB) in pain modulation is well documented (Fuentes et al. 1999). Administration of anandamide, Δ^9-tetrahydrocannabinoid (Δ^9-THC), and various selective CB receptor agonists, have shown antinociceptive effects in a variety of acute (Buxbaum 1972; Welch and Stevens 1992) and chronic (Sofia et al. 1973; Smith et al. 1998) models of nociception (for review see Pertwee 2001). These antinociceptive effects are mediated by CB1 receptors located at spinal (Yaksh 1981; Lichtman and Martin 1991; Welsh and Stevens 1992) and supraspinal sites (Lichtman and Martin 1991; Martin et al. 1993) as well as CB1 (Richardson et al. 1998) and CB2 receptors (Jagger et al. 1998) located in peripheral tissues (for review see Pertwee 2001). Although numerous studies suggest otherwise (Onaivi et al. 1990; McGregor et al. 1996; Sanudo-Pena et al. 1997; Tzschentke 1998), several experiments implicate cannabinoid systems in reward. For example, Δ^9-THC is self administered in humans (Chait and Burke 1994) and squirrel monkeys (Tanda et al. 2000), lowers intracranial self-stimulation thresholds in rats (Gardner et al. 1988) and produces place preference in rats (Lepore et al. 1995). Δ^9-THC has been shown to increase firing of dopamine neurons in the nucleus accumbens (Gessa et al. 1998), as well as increase dopamine levels in the shell of the nucleus accumbens (Tanda et al. 1997). Collectively, these studies suggest that CB reinforcement is likely mediated through the same mesolimbic dopaminergic systems involved in opioid and psychostimulant reward (Koob and Bloom 1988). While one literature clearly suggests CB receptors present a viable target for analgesic drugs (for review see Pertwee 2001), a second literature suggests these putative analgesic compounds are likely to possess an abuse liability (Gessa et al. 1998).

Recent research indicates that the use of certain analgesics (e.g., morphine) that possess several liabilities (tolerance, dependence, etc.) may not be as controversial as previously suggested. Rats given repeated administration of morphine in the context of formalin-induced inflammatory nociception displayed less tolerance to morphine (Vaccarino et al. 1993; Bardin et al. 2000) and less severe withdrawal symptoms in response to a naloxone challenge (Vaccarino and Couret 1993; Bardin et al. 2000). In addition, rats given repeated administration of morphine in the context of chronic inflammatory pain induced by complete Freund's adjuvant (CFA) developed tolerance at slower rates and showed lower incidences of naloxone precipitated withdrawal symptoms (Lerida et al. 1987). Similar findings on tolerance and dependence have been observed clinically with opioid therapies (for review see Melzak 1991). Long-term use of codeine and oxycodone for chronic rheumatic conditions significantly reduced pain without requiring increased dosing except in cases where a worsening of the painful condition existed (Ytterberg et al. 1998). Collectively, these data suggest the liabilities of analgesics may be greatly reduced when these compounds are used in the context of pain management.

The medical use of cannabis for the treatment of chronic pain remains highly controversial. However, this controversy may be obviated by the development of the pro-drug Δ^9-THC hemisuccinate (Δ^9-THC-HS) and its formulation as a suppository (Mattes et al. 1993). This formulation is but one solution to the undesirable inhalation route of cannabis administration. Moreover, rectal administration of Δ^9-THC-HS has been shown to produce a pharmacokinetic profile that is highly desirable for putative therapeutic agents. First, blood levels of Δ^9-THC and other CB metabolites do not show the rapid elevation typical of the inhalation route, which is commonly associated with euphoric effects. Second, blood levels of these constituents remain relatively stable for up to 6-8 hrs post administration (for review, see Walker et al. 1999). These pharmacokinetic factors, along with the notion that context is important in drug responses, suggest that Δ^9-THC-HS may not possess the reinforcing properties when administered in the context of chronic pain. To explore this possibility, the present study examined the antinociceptive as well as the rewarding properties of Δ^9-THC-HS in the complete Freund's adjuvant (CFA) model of chronic inflammatory pain.

METHOD

Place Preference Test

The conditioned place preference (CPP) paradigm (for review see Carr et al. 1989) is a procedure that is commonly used to evaluate the reinforcing and aversive properties of drugs (van der Kooy 1987). This paradigm is based on traditional learning principles and involves the pairing of a drug state with environments having distinctive stimuli (i.e., place). Following several drug-place pairings, an animal's preference is ascertained by examining approach responses to and maintenance of contact with the drug-paired environment. The CPP paradigm has become a frequently used method in behavioral pharmacology for examination of the positively reinforcing properties of abused drugs.

Male Lewis strain rats (100-125 g; Harlan, Indianapolis, IN) were housed in suspended steel cages (360 cm^2), maintained under a 12 hour light/dark cycle in a temperature controlled vivarium (22 ± 1°C). Food and water were available *ad lib*. After a one-week acclimation period, animals received one week of handling exposure to reduce experimenter-related stress. Research protocols were approved by the Institutional Animal Care and Use Committee and were conducted under the ethical guidelines of the International Association for the Study of Pain (Zimmerman 1983).

The groups in this study formed a 2 × 3 factorial design that combined 2 levels of inflammation (CFA inflamed vs. non-inflamed) with 3 levels of drug (0.0, 2.5, or 5.0 mg/kg Δ^9-THC-HS). Sample sizes were n = 7 per group. Persistent unilateral inflammation was produced by injections of 0.1 ml of complete Freund's adjuvant (CFA: Sigma; St. Louis, MO) into the left hind paw (Butler et al. 1992). This model of arthritis produces long-lasting inflammation leading to hyperalgesia and joint destruction and bony proliferation of the metatarsal, tarsal, and ankle regions. Non-inflamed control rats did not receive this explicit manipulation. CFA was administered several hours after acclimation to the place preference apparatus.

Δ^9-THC-HS (5 mg/kg/ml) or vehicle (Wacbee W) was administered immediately before the start of each conditioning trial (see below). Compounds were melted (45°C) prior to rectal administration to obviate the possibility of the animal evacuating a solid suppository. Pilot data examining plasma levels at various time points of rectal administration of melted Δ^9-THC-HS show that peak plasma Δ^9-THC levels were detected at 15 min post administration (approximately 110 ng/ml). This was followed by a gradual decline in plasma Δ^9-THC levels at 30 min (40 ng/ml); relatively stable Δ^9-THC levels were detected from between 60-360 min post-administration (15-25 ng/ml).

Six T-shaped place preference chambers were used in this study (see Sufka and Roach 1996 for details). The place preference procedure involved three phases consisting of one apparatus acclimation trial, eight drug/vehicle conditioning trials, and six discrete choice trials. The acclimation trial allowed animal access to the entire apparatus for a 15 min period one day before conditioning trials. The eight conditioning trials (1 per day of 60 minutes) consisted of counter-balanced, alternate-day pairings of drug (0.0, 2.5 and 5.0 mg/kg/ml) with the white compartment and vehicle (0.0) with the black compartment for a total of four pairings each. Drug preference was determined by the animal's choice behavior (i.e., first entry) to the drug-paired (white) vs. vehicle-paired (black) compartment on six discrete preference trials conducted two per day over a three day period and were conducted under drug-free states. From these choice measures, a single preference score was derived using the following formula: Preference Score = number of white compartment entries/6 (Sufka 1994).

Hotplate Test

Tests of thermal nociception were conducted on the fourth day of drug exposure (Day 7 or 8 of conditioning trials). Rats were removed from the conditioning apparatus and placed on a hotplate apparatus with a surface temperature maintained at 50°C. Latency to lick a hind-paw served as the dependent measure. Animals that failed to exhibit a lick response in 30 seconds were removed from the hotplate and assigned a latency score of 30 seconds. Animals were euthanized at the conclusion of the experiment.

RESULTS

Δ^9-THC-HS effects on thermal nociception are summarized in Figure 1.

Adjuvant-inflamed rats exhibited shorter response latencies than non-inflamed rats under the drug vehicle condition (i.e., hyperalgesia). In general, Δ^9-THC-HS increased latency scores for both groups compared to respective controls. A 2-way ANOVA revealed a significant main effect of inflammation $F(1,36) = 31.44$, $p = 0.0001$ and a significant drug effect $F(2,36) = 3.980$, $p = 0.03$. The inflammation $\times$ drug interaction term was not significant. Post hoc comparisons using Fisher's PLSD detected significantly shorter latency scores for CFA-inflamed animals compared to non-inflamed animals under vehicle condition ($p < 0.05$) (hyperalgesia). Further analyses revealed a significant increase in latency scores for the 5.0 mg/kg non-inflamed group compared to

FIGURE 1. Mean hotplate latency ($\pm$SEM) as a function of Δ^9-THC-HS dose for CFA-inflamed and non-inflamed animals.

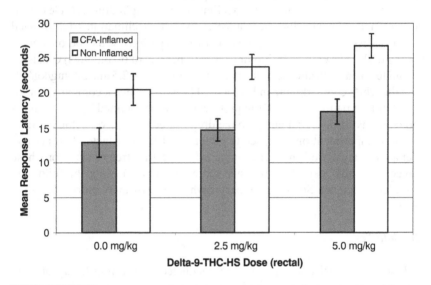

HOTPLATE DATA

	Inflamed	Non-Inflamed
	Mean	Mean
0.0 mg/kg	12.90	20.49
2.5 mg/kg	14.71	23.74
5.0 mg/kg	17.32	26.77
	SE	SE
0.0 mg/kg	2.11	2.27
2.5 mg/kg	1.59	1.78
5.0 mg/kg	1.80	1.75

non-inflamed controls ($p < 0.05$). Although there was a trend in CFA-inflamed latency scores, no significant differences were observed. No further analyses were conducted on these data.

Δ^9-THC-HS effects on preference scores for CFA-inflamed and non-inflamed animals are summarized in Figure 2.

Both groups showed a black compartment bias under the no drug condition. In general, Δ^9-THC-HS produced a dose dependent increase in preference scores in non-inflamed animals. However, this pattern was not seen in CFA-inflamed animals. Consistent with these observations, a 2-way ANOVA revealed a significant main effect for inflammation, $F(1,36) = 7.353$, $p = 0.01$, no

FIGURE 2. Mean preference scores (±SEM) as a function of Δ^9-THC-HS dose for CFA-inflamed and non-inflamed animals.

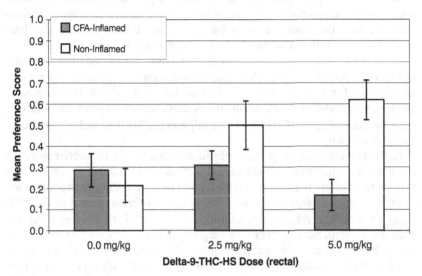

CPP DATA

	Inflamed	Non-Inflamed
	Mean	Mean
0.0 mg/kg	0.29	0.21
2.5 mg/kg	0.31	0.50
5.0 mg/kg	0.17	0.62
	SE	SE
0.0 mg/kg	0.08	0.08
2.5 mg/kg	0.07	0.12
5.0 mg/kg	0.07	0.09

main effect for drug, and a significant inflammation $\times$ drug interaction, $F(2,36) = 4.634$, $p < 0.02$. Post hoc comparisons using Fisher's PLSD established no significant difference in baseline preference scores, indicating that the bias was present regardless of inflammation condition. Further post hoc analyses revealed a significant increase in preference scores for non-inflamed animals at the 2.5 and 5.0 mg/kg doses compared to vehicle controls ($p < 0.05$), indicative of cannabinoid positive reinforcement in these animals. However, for adjuvant-inflamed groups, preference scores were unaffected by Δ^9-THC-HS, suggesting that Δ^9-THC-HS lacks positively reinforcing properties in the context of persistent inflammatory pain.

DISCUSSION

While CB receptors present a viable target for pain management, the therapeutic use of cannabinoids remains controversial. However, an emerging literature suggests that analgesic drug liabilities can be diminished when these compounds are utilized in the context of pain management. These observations, along with the highly desirable pharmacokinetic profile of the suppository formulation of Δ^9-THC-HS, suggest that certain cannabinoids may provide for pain relief in some settings with little addictive liabilities. The purpose of the present research was to examine the putative antinociceptive and reinforcing properties of Δ^9-THC-HS in the rat adjuvant arthritis model of chronic inflammatory pain.

In the present study, adjuvant arthritic animals displayed shorter response latencies to a noxious thermal stimulus than non-inflamed controls. This hyperalgesic effect is consistent with reports of long lasting changes in nociceptive responses associated with CFA-induced arthritis (Lewis et al. 1985; Butler et al. 1992). While rectal administration of Δ^9-THC-HS tended to produce a dose-dependent increase in response latencies in both inflamed and non-inflamed groups, this antinociceptive effect was significant in only the non-inflamed animals. These findings are consistent with reports of cannabinoid modulation of thermal nociception in acute models (Buxbaum 1972; Yaksh 1981; Welch and Stevens 1992), but inconsistent with reports of cannabinoid modulation of hyperalgesia in chronic inflammatory models (Sofia et al. 1973; Smith et al. 1998). However, recent research suggests that cannabinoid agonists may be more effective in preventing the development of hyperalgesia than attenuating it (Li et al. 1999a). It is also possible that higher doses of Δ^9-THC-HS are required to modulate the thermal hyperalgesia in this CFA model of chronic inflammation. Finally, subsequent power analyses assuming a large effect size indicated that a significant analgesic effect would have been detected at the 5.0 mg dose in inflamed animals with the addition of as few as 7 animals per cell.

In the conditioned place preference test, both non-inflamed and CFA-inflamed animals that received vehicle in both conditioning compartments displayed a black compartment preference (i.e., preference scores under 0.5). This is not an unexpected finding and it is the principle reason for pairing all drug conditioning trials with the white compartment (i.e., condition against a black compartment preference). These baseline preference scores in vehicle-treated animals did not differ significantly between inflammation groups.

In non-inflamed animals, rectal administration of Δ^9-THC-HS produced a significant dose-dependent increase in place preference scores, a pattern of effects indicative of reward (for reviews see van der Kooy, 1987; Carr et al. 1989). These findings add to a literature that is considered equivocal at best on the reinforcing properties of cannabinoids (see Tzschentke 1998 for review). For example, Mallet and Beninger (1998) report that in Wistar rats anandamide failed to produce place preference while Δ^9-THC produced place aversion. Place aversion has also been reported in Lister hooded rats using either CB receptor agonists or Δ^9-THC (Cheer et al. 2000). In contrast, cannabinoids produce place preference (when using a similar procedure and comparable doses) in Long Evans rats (Lepore et al. 1995), are self-administered in squirrel monkeys (Tanda et al. 2000) and produce lower thresholds for intracranial self stimulation in Lewis strain rats (Gardner et al. 1988). While the use of various animal models and paradigms may contribute to such equivocal findings, a growing literature suggests that strain differences in drug sensitivity may be an equally important methodological consideration (for review see Mogil 1999). Lepore et al. (1996) report that in an intracranial self stimulation paradigm, Lewis rats, which we used in the present study, are much more responsive to the rewarding properties of Δ^9-THC compared to Fischer 344 and Sprague-Dawley rats.

In contrast to non-inflamed groups, CFA-inflamed animals given rectal Δ^9-THC-HS did not show significant changes in their place preference scores, a finding that suggests an absence of drug reward in these groups. This finding is somewhat surprising in light of studies that demonstrate analgesic drugs produce place preference though their negative reinforcing properties (i.e., pain reduction) in models of chronic pain (Sufka 1994; Sufka and Roach 1996). However, one requirement for an analgesic drug to possess negative reinforcing properties is that it be sufficiently potent in reducing inflammatory nociception. While rectal administration of Δ^9-THC-HS significantly affected thermal nociception in non-inflamed animals, it was only modestly analgesic in attenuating thermal hyperalgesia in the CFA model of chronic inflammation and, therefore may not possess the necessary negatively reinforcing properties to support place preference. Given that Δ^9-THC-HS does not possess the same reinforcing properties in inflamed groups as it does in non-inflamed controls, we suggest that context can be an important determinant in drug responses.

To our knowledge, this is the first study assessing both the analgesic and reinforcing properties of cannabinoids in the context of chronic pain. While the finding that animals in persistent pain show less analgesia and reward have been interpreted by some to suggest accelerated tolerance (Gutstein et al. 1995; Li et al. 1999b), this interpretation is unlikely. Animals in the present study received low doses of Δ^9-THC-HS and on alternate day exposures, a procedure highly unlikely to produce tolerance. A more likely explanation is that the context in which drugs are employed is an important determinant in drug effects. Bardin et al. (2000, p. 61) have suggested, "that theories of (opiate) tolerance, withdrawal, and reward should incorporate the effects of pain." For example, opioid agonists given repeatedly in the context of persistent or chronic pain show reduced tolerance, physical dependence and withdrawal while maintaining analgesic efficacy (Lerida et al. 1987; Vaccarino and Couret 1993; Vaccarino et al. 1993). The results of the present study are consistent with these findings and extend the importance of context to include cannabinoid systems and reward behaviors. Further studies evaluating therapeutic compounds should consider the context as an important determinant in drug response.

AUTHOR NOTE

This research was supported in part by The National Center for Natural Products Research and ElSohly Laboratories, Inc. The authors would like to thank Jamie Neal, Brad Sheals, and Sarah Hoffman for assisting in data collection.

REFERENCES

Bardin L., J.A. Kim, S. Siegal, 2000. The role of formalin-induced pain in morphine tolerance, withdrawal, and reward. *Exp Clin Psychopharmacol* 8:61-67.
Butler, S.H., F. Godefroy, J.M. Besson, J. Weil-Fugazza, 1992. A limited arthritic model for chronic pain studies in the rat. *Pain* 48:73-81.
Buxbaum, D.M. 1972. Analgesic activity of Δ^9-tetrahydrocannabinol in the rat and mouse. *Psychopharmacologia* 25:275-280.
Carr, G.D., H.C. Fibiger, A.G. Phillips. 1989. *Conditioned place preference as a measure of drug reward*. In: J.M. Liebman and S.J. Cooper (Eds.), *The Neuropharmacological Basis of Reward*. Clarendon Press: Oxford. pp. 264-319.
Chait, L.D., K.A. Burke. 1994. Preference for high-versus low-potency marijuana. *Pharmacol Biochem Behav* 49:643-647.
Cheer, J.F, D.A. Kendall, C.A. Marsden. 2000. Cannabinoid receptors and reward in the rat: a conditioned place preference study. *Psychopharmacology (Berl)* 151(1): 25-30.
Fuentes J.A., M. Ruiz-Gayo, J. Manzanares, G. Vela, I. Reche, J. Corchero. 1999. Cannabinoids as potential new analgesics. *Life Sci* 65:675-685.
Gardner, E.L., W. Paredes, D. Smith, A. Donner, C. Milling, and D. Morrison. 1988. Facilitation of brain stimulation reward by Δ^9-tetrahydrocannabinol. *Psychopharmacol* 96:142-144.
Gardner, E.L., S.R. Vorel. 1998. Cannabinoid transmission and reward-related events. *Neurobiol Dis* 5(6 Pt B):502-533.
Gessa, G.L., M. Melis, A.L. Muntoni, M. Diana. 1998. Cannabinoids activate mesolimbic dopamine neurons by an action on cannabinoid CB_1 receptors. *Eur J Pharmacol* 341:39-44.
Gutstein, H.B., K.A. Trujillo, H. Akil. 1995. Does chronic nociceptive stimulation alter the development of morphine tolerance? *Brain Res* 680:174-179.

Jagger, S.I., F.S. Hasnie, S. Sellaturay, A.S.C. Rice. 1998. The anti-hyperalgesic actions of the cannabinoid anandamide and the putative CB2 receptor agonist palmitoylethanolamide in visceral and somatic inflammatory pain. *Pain* 76:189-199.

Koob, G.F., F.E. Bloom. 1988. Cellular and molecular mechanisms of drug dependence. *Science* 242:715-723.

Lepore, M., X. Liu, V. Savage, D. Matalon, E.L. Gardner. 1996. Genetic differences in delta-9-tetrahydrocannabinol-induced facilitation of brain stimulation reward as measured by a rate-frequency curve-shift electrical brain stimulation paradigm in three different rat strains. *Life Sci* 58(25):PL365-72.

Lepore, M., S.R. Vorel, J. Lowinson, E.L. Gardner. 1995. Conditioned place preference induced by Δ^9-tetrahydrocannabinol: comparison with cocaine, morphine, and food reward. *Life Sci* 56(23,24):2073-2080.

Lerida, M., P. Sanchez-Blazquez, J. Garzon. 1987. Incidence of morphine withdrawal and quasi-abstinence syndrome in a model of chronic pain in the rat. *Neurosci Lett* 81:155-158.

Lewis, A.J., R.P. Carlson, J. Chang. 1985. Experimental models of inflammation. In: I.L. Bonta, M.A. Bray, and M.J. Parnham (Eds.). *The Pharmacology of Inflammation (Handbook of Inflammation*, vol 5). New York: Elsevier. pp. 371-397.

Li, J.Y., R.S. Daughters, C. Bullis, R. Bengiamin, M.W. Stucky, J. Brennan, D.A. Simone. 1999a. The cannabinoid receptor agonist WIN 55,212-2 mesylate blocks the development of hyperalgesia produced by capsaicin in rats. *Pain* 81:25-33.

Li, J.Y., C.H. Wong, K.S. Huang, K.W. Liang, M. L. Lin, P.P. Tan, J.C. Chen. 1999b. Morphine tolerance in arthritic rats and serotonergic system. *Life Sci* 64(10): PL111-116.

Lichtman, A.H., B.R. Martin. 1991. Spinal and supraspinal components of cannabinoid-induced antinociception. *J Pharmacol Exper Therap* 258:517-523.

Mallet, P.E., R.J. Beninger. 1998. Delta-9-tetrahydrocannabinol, but not the endogenous cannabinoid receptor ligand anandamide, produces conditioned place avoidance. *Life Sci* 62(26):2431-2439.

Martin, B.J., N.K. Lai, K.T. Patrick, J.M. Walker. 1993. Antinociceptive actions of cannabinoids following intraventricular administration in rats. *Brain Res* 629: 300-304.

Mattes, R.D., L.M. Shaw, J. Edling-Owens, K. Engelman, M.A. ElSohly. 1993. Bypassing the first-pass effect for the therapeutic use of cannabinoids. *Pharmacol Biochem Behav* 44:745-747.

McGregor, I.S., C.N. Issakidis, G. Prior. 1996. Aversive effects of the synthetic cannabinoid CP 55,940 in rats. *Pharmacol Biochem Behav* 53(3):657-664.

Melzack, R. 1991. The tragedy of needless pain. *Sci Am* 262:27-33.

Mogil, J.S. 1999. The genetic mediation of individual differences in sensitivity to pain and its inhibition. *Proc Natl Acad Sci* 96(14):7744-7751.

Onaivi, E.S., M.R. Green, B.R. Martin. 1990. Pharmacological characterization of cannabinoids in the elevated plus maze. *J Pharmacol Exper Therap* 253:1002-1009.

Pertwee, R.G. 2001. Cannabinoid receptors and pain. *Progr Neurobiol* 63:569-611.

Richardson, J.D., S. Kilo, K.M. Hargreaves. 1998. Cannabinoids reduce hyperalgesia and inflammation via interaction with peripheral CB_1 receptors. *Pain* 75:111-119.

Sanudo-Pena, M.C., K. Tsou, E.R. Delay, A.G. Hohman, M. Force, J.M. Walker. 1997. Endogenous cannabinoids as an aversive or counter-rewarding system in the rat. *Neurosci Lett* 223(2):125-128.

Smith, L., K. Fujimori, J. Lowe, S. Welch. 1998. Characterization of Δ^9-tetrahydrocannabinal and anandamide antinociception in nonarthritic and arthritic rats. *Pharmacol Biochem Behav* 60:183-191.

Sofia R.D., S.D. Nalepa, J.J. Harakal, H.B. Vassar. 1973. Anti-edema and analgesic properties of Δ^9-tetrahydrocannabinal (THC). *J Pharmacol Exper Therap* 186: 646-655.

Sufka, K.J. 1994. Conditioned place preference paradigm: a novel approach for analgesic drug assessment against chronic pain. *Pain* 58:355-366.

Sufka, K.J., J.T. Roach. 1996. Stimulus properties and antinociceptive effects of selective bradykinin B_1 and B_2 receptor antagonists in rats. *Pain* 66:99-103.

Tanda, G., P. Munzar, S.R. Goldberg. 2000. Self-administration behavior is maintained by the psychoactive ingredient of marijuana in squirrel monkeys. *Nature Neurosci* 3:1073-1074.

Tanda, G., F.E. Pontieri, G. Di Chiara. 1997. Cannabinoid and heroin activation of mesolimbic dopamine transmission by a common μ_1 opioid receptor mechanism. *Science* 276:2048-2049.

Tzschentke, T.M. 1998. Measuring reward with the conditioned place preference paradigm: A comprehensive review of drug effects. Recent progress and new issues. *Progr Neurobiol* 56:613-672.

Vaccarino, A.L., P. Marek, B. Kest, S. Ben-Eliyahu, L.C. Couret Jr, B. Kao, J.C. Liebeskind. 1993. Morphine fails to produce tolerance when administered in the presence of formalin pain in rats. *Brain Res* 627(2):287-290.

Vaccarino, A.L., L.C. Couret Jr. 1993. Formalin-induced pain antagonizes the development of opiate dependence in the rat. *Neurosci Lett* 161(2):195-198.

van der Kooy, D. 1987. Place conditioning: a simple and effective method for assessing the motivational properties of drugs. In: M.A. Bozarth (Ed.), *Method for assessing the Reinforcing properties of Abused drugs*. New York: Spring. pp. 229-240.

Walker, L.A., E.C. Harland, A.M. Best, M.A. ElSohly. 1999. Δ^9-THC hemisuccinate in suppository form as an alternative to oral and smoked THC. In: G.G. Nahas, K.M. Sutin, and D.J. Harvey (eds.). *Marihuana and Medicine*. Totowa, NJ: Humana Press, pp. 123-135.

Welch, S.P., D.L. Stevens. 1992. Antinociceptive activity of intrathecally administered cannabinoids alone, and in combination with morphine, in mice. *J Pharmacol Exper Therap* 262:10-18.

Yaksh, T.L. 1981. The antinociceptive effects of intrathecally administered levonantradol and desacetyllevonantradol in the rat. *J Clin Pharmacol* 21:334s-340s.

Ytterberg, S.R., M.L. Mahowald, S.R. Woods. 1998. Codeine and oxycodone use in patients with chronic rheumatic disease pain. *Arthritis Rheum* 41(9):1603-1612.

Zimmerman, M. 1983. Ethical guidelines for investigations of experimental pain in conscious animals. *Pain* 16:109-110.

Prospects for New Cannabis-Based Prescription Medicines

Brian A. Whittle
Geoffrey W. Guy
Philip Robson

SUMMARY. Cannabis is now emerging from a period of prohibition and being revisited as a potential source of treatments for conditions ill served by synthetic substances. Previous research focussed primarily on effects produced by synthetic cannabinoids such as THC, or cannabis of unknown cannabinoid content. Chemovars of cannabis characterized by high content of specific cannabinoids (primarily, but not only THC and CBD) have been developed. Clinical research using defined extracts from these chemovars is now underway in the UK.

Many diseases are multifactorial; a variety of receptors need to be targeted to produce a therapeutic effect. A defined botanical may better achieve this than a single synthetic compound as the components can act synergistically. A new generation of cannabis based medicinal products takes advantage of increasing understanding of the mode of action of cannabinoids, evidence-based research on clinical uses and new technology for realization of products, in anti-diversionary presentations. *[Article copies available for a fee from The Haworth Document Delivery Service: 1-800-342-9678. E-mail address: <getinfo@haworthpressinc.com> Website: <http://www.HaworthPress.com> © 2001 by The Haworth Press, Inc. All rights reserved.]*

Brian A. Whittle, Geoffrey W. Guy and Philip Robson are affiliated with GW Pharmaceuticals Ltd., Porton Down Science Park, Salisbury, Wiltshire, UK SP4 0JQ.

[Haworth co-indexing entry note]: "Prospects for New Cannabis-Based Prescription Medicines." Whittle, Brian A., Geoffrey W. Guy, and Philip Robson. Co-published simultaneously in *Journal of Cannabis Therapeutics* (The Haworth Integrative Healing Press, an imprint of The Haworth Press, Inc.) Vol. 1, No. 3/4, 2001, pp. 183-205; and: *Cannabis Therapeutics in HIV/AIDS* (ed: Ethan Russo) The Haworth Integrative Healing Press, an imprint of The Haworth Press, Inc., 2001, pp. 183-205. Single or multiple copies of this article are available for a fee from The Haworth Document Delivery Service [1-800-342-9678, 9:00 a.m. - 5:00 p.m. (EST). E-mail address: getinfo@haworthpressinc.com].

KEYWORDS. Cannabinoids, cannabis, CB receptors, new chemovars, clinical research, multiple sclerosis, spinal cord injury, neurogenic pain, botanical extracts, secure dispensing, alternative delivery systems, harm reduction

PROSPECTS FOR NEW CANNABIS-BASED PRESCRIPTION MEDICINES

There is nothing new about cannabis as a prescription medicine. The use of cannabis by mankind is probably as old as the need for pain relief but the use of cannabis as a prescription medicine is complicated by its alternate use as a recreational drug, and attempts to regulate that practice. The novelty described in this article arises from a re-examination of some historical uses of cannabis in the light of new technology. Research on possible modes of action of cannabinoids, and novel methods of administration have prompted a re-evaluation of the therapeutic benefit of cannabis and cannabinoids.

A distinction has to be made between the cultivation of hemp, which is primarily used for textile fibre and oil seed on the one hand, and cannabis, which is used for medicinal purposes on the other. Botanists are still debating whether *Cannabis sativa* and *Cannabis indica* are two species within the family Cannabaceae, or whether there is only one species with great diversity. The various uses of *Cannabis* spp. arise from crosses and selective breeding of varieties from various landraces. The plasticity of the cannabis genome provides opportunities for rational investigation of cannabis by providing defined chemovars. The availability of specific chemovars (varieties distinguished by the active constituents which they contain rather than fine differences in morphology) provides the test materials to cater for the current resurgence of interest in the therapeutic benefit of cannabis-based medicines.

The first edition of Merck's Manual (1899) reflects the important place that cannabis-based medicines had in the armamentarium of physicians at that time. At the end of the 19th century the majority of active drug substances were *materia medica* of plant origin. It is interesting that cannabis-based medicines provided treatments for conditions which, during the pharmaceutical revolution over the last half-century, have come to be catered for by synthetic drugs such as the benzodiazepines and potent synthetic analgesics. In Merck's Manual, preparations of cannabis are recommended as a hypnotic sedative which is very useful for the treatment of hysteria, delirium, epilepsy, nervous insomnia, migraine, pain and dysmenorrhoea. It is worth remembering that at that time, the available hypnotics were bromides, extracts of valerian and opium. Apparently, extracts of cannabis were prescribed for Queen Victoria, and in Victorian times, cannabis was a respectable and useful component of prescribed medicines. It continued in use until the middle of the 20th Century but social abuse caused a re-think on the risks perceived to attend its use. Its use as a prescription medicine was reduced and finally prohibited by legislation.

The renewal of interest in cannabis-based medicines may lead to treatments for conditions which cannot be adequately treated by the best available medicines based on synthetic compounds. It is therefore vital that introduction of cannabis-based medicines is justified on the grounds of evidence-based medicine.

The use of cannabis as a recreational substance has resulted in the classification of cannabis as a Schedule I drug in the USA. Corresponding proscriptive legislation has been enacted by other signatories to the United Nations Single Convention. This reflects the regulatory attitude that it is a drug of potential abuse with no therapeutic benefit. In order to show that cannabis-based medicines have therapeutic benefit it is necessary to carry out clinical research. In order to carry out clinical research it is necessary to have a license to possess cannabis for research purposes. Although such licensing is theoretically possible, it has not until now been considered expedient to support research into the clinical usefulness of cannabis. Since 1971, the type of research that has received most support in the USA has been directed towards demonstrating the risks and hazards of taking marijuana. Research into its therapeutic benefit has not been practically possible or politically correct until very recently.

The House of Lords Science and Technology Sub Committee report (2001) gave very positive encouragement to carry out clinical research in the UK. With the support of the UK Home Office and the Medicines Control Agency (MCA) clinical research is now underway in the UK in patients with pain and associated with Multiple Sclerosis (MS), other neuropathic pain, and cancer pain unresponsive to opioids.

During the last three decades the main avenues of research have been pre-clinical investigations into the mode of action of cannabinoids and cannabinoid-like compounds. Clinical research has focused on the effects (mostly adverse events), which follow from use of marijuana either in smoked or orally ingested form. The majority of work on cannabis in the USA has employed a variety of cannabis that contains delta-9 tetrahydrocannabinol (THC) as the principle cannabinoid. In America and the Caribbean, there has been selection of plant varieties that produce maximum psychotropic effects, and this material contains only a small proportion of cannabidiol (CBD). In contrast, street material in Europe contains proportionately more CBD (about equal quantities of THC and CBD). This type of cannabis is referred to as "Moroccan"; it is grown in many European and Mediterranean countries.

Cannabidiol was formerly regarded as an inactive constituent of cannabis (Merck Index 1996), but there is now evidence that it has pharmacological activity, which is different from that of THC in several respects. In some cases it appears that the pharmacological effects are different in sign, and that a combination of the two cannabinoids has therapeutic benefit not evidenced by either cannabinoid alone. In the case of cannabis there is evidence from clinical studies, and a strong patient perception that the ceiling of effect produced by extracts is greater than the effect produced by the corresponding amount of THC as a pure chemical substance (Price and Notcutt 1998).

In a regulatory climate where the emphasis is on new chemical entities, it is refreshing to see that the idea of using cannabis as a "botanical" extract is attracting serious attention. It means that clinical investigators can use a defined extract rather than a mixture of synthetic cannabinoids as the test object. Many of the reports of early work on cannabis are based on observations of subjects who smoked marijuana. Unfortunately, in the majority of these reports a clear understanding of the content of the major cannabinoids is lacking. The availability of cannabis with a pedigree and provenance allows for this variable to be controlled rigorously.

There are therefore a number of issues that need to be addressed in rehabilitating cannabis, first of all for some of its historic indications, and also for newer indications especially those areas where cannabis has a unique contribution. Among these are its use in the field of opioid-resistant pain in neurological conditions such as multiple sclerosis, cancer pain and migraine, and as an appetite stimulant in AIDS syndrome. In order to do this it is necessary to revisit the regulatory and statutory requirements for cannabis-based medicines. The major issues are:

- the concept of cannabis-based medicines as botanicals as opposed to pure cannabinoids;
- selective breeding of high yielding chemovars that produce an abundance of one particular cannabinoid;
- investigation of the pharmacological properties of various cannabinoids, i.e., cannabis is not just THC;
- variability of composition of cannabis. The geographical and genetic basis for variation in cannabinoid content of cannabis biomass and its control to give a standardized product;
- the quality aspects of cannabis biomass production;
- routes of administration and optimization of formulations to achieve particular pharmacokinetic profiles;
- regulatory issues, including health registration, and international legal requirements;
- security packaging and anti-diversionary devices which can be used in connection with cannabis-based medicines in order to satisfy statutory requirements.

THE RATIONALE FOR USE OF CANNABIS EXTRACTS

The pharmaceutical revolution in the 20th Century has been built on the concept of treating disease as a target that can be hit with a defined chemical compound. The discovery of receptors in tissues to which drugs bind, and in which they initiate a biological effect gave support to this idea. It is ironic that the concept of the "magic bullet" came to be understood in terms of targeting "receptors." With the advent of cloned receptor proteins it is now possible to show that a variety of targets may need to be hit in order to effect a therapeutic benefit. It seems likely that what is needed is a broadside rather than a sniper's bullet to despatch the pathological lesion. It is true that some diseases are the result of a single biochemical defect, for example the congenital absence of a particular enzyme system in phenylketuronia, but the majority of disease processes are multifactorial and have to be tackled holistically. Pathological lesions, where they can be considered as causative, require a number of therapeutic agents, or a single chemical with several properties, to achieve an improvement in the patient's condition. Plants contain a variety of active and adjuvant substances, and by a process of selection those that are clinically beneficial have become accepted as *materia medica*. Humans have been exposed to these complex mixtures for millennia. Those that are useful have been selected, and it is hypothesized that they present less of a metabolic shock than synthetic new chemical entities. In practice it has been found that extracts of cannabis provide greater relief of pain than the equivalent amount of cannabinoid given as a single chemical entity.

POLYPHARMACY

In medical education over the last half century, polypharmacy has been frowned upon. It was considered desirable in an age when new chemical entities were discovered with precise effects on biological systems and even particular receptors that these "clean" chemicals could be used to treat pathological lesions with surgical precision. Unfortunately, human disease has multiple pathologies and is rarely treatable with a single chemical agent. By default, a number of new chemical entities are used in order to treat different aspects of the patient's condition holistically. In plant extracts accessory constituents may produce an effect that is synergistic with the principal one. Others may mitigate side effects produced by one drug. By repeated use and empirical observation, these processes have selected the *materia medica* that are most useful and safe. Polypharmacy is a defining characteristic of most systems of traditional medicine, but it is sometimes overlooked that combination of agents in complex prescriptions was common in the UK until the third quarter of the 20th Century. The reasons for using combinations of *materia medica* as active ingredients in Western prescriptions were four-fold. The prescription typically contained a principal active ingredient, a secondary ingredient, which was thought to have an adjuvant effect, a substance that antagonized some of the adverse events, and excipients, which had a physical function in ensuring the stability and patient acceptability of the total prescription. This style of prescription was phased out in the second half of the 20th Century, with the end of extemporaneous dispensing in the UK. However, when a botanical extract is tested in a well designed trial it is possible to justify clinical research on the extract as it is. It may contain more than one active ingredient. However, if it is presented as a well-defined botanical drug it can be used as a drug substance in its own right. The requirements from a regulatory point of view are that the medication should have the same composition each time it is prepared and be stable. In the case of cannabis, the limited stability of some of the older galenic preparations may have been a factor in their falling out of use. Improved methods of selection of plants, care in growing and improved methods of analysis now provide materials which can be used confidently as drug substances in their own right.

EFFICACY

Mechoulam (1976) showed that many of the characteristic effects of cannabis are produced by Δ^9-tetrahydrocannabinol. The availability of synthetic THC prompted the investigation of this chemical entity as the active ingredient in pharmaceutical preparations. Dronabinol (Marinol®) is available as soft gelatin capsules containing 2.5, 5 and 10 mg of THC. As a synthetic compound it falls outside the Single Convention on Narcotics and is available as a prescription medicine. It has been progressively moved from schedule I and is now in Schedule III. Dronabinol capsules have an indication as an anti-emetic and have also been shown to stimulate appetite in patients with AIDS. The oral route of administration for cannabinoids leads to slow and irregular absorption. Some of the variability in response and low therapeutic window may be inevitable consequences of giving the drug by this route. Perhaps of greater significance is the pharmacokinetic profile after administration. Once the capsule is swallowed it is committed, and one of the unfortunate adverse events following the use of Marinol® is that the patients who are heavily sedated ('stoned'), have to wait until the effect wears off. Comparisons of the effect of preparations containing dronabinol with those containing an equivalent amount of THC in the form of a cannabis extract (Iversen 2000) have shown that the maximal therapeutic effect and incidence of adverse events is lower when the cannabinoid is given as extract.

A number of explanations have been offered for the lower incidence of side effects and the higher ceiling of cannabis extracts over synthetic cannabinoids. In cannabis-based medicines, the presence of other cannabinoids such as cannabidiol (CBD) is thought to have an antagonistic effect to some of the effects of THC, although CBD may sum with other THC effects. The basis for this explanation is illustrated in Table 1, which shows, in broad outline, the different pharmacological effects of THC and CBD. It is clear from this table that all of the effects of cannabis cannot be explained in terms of just one cannabinoid. It is equally true that combination of THC and CBD in the correct proportions can offer a product with a tailored pharmacological and therapeutic profile, and possibly a lower cost in terms of adverse events.

In a pilot pharmacological screening test (In-house report, GPA 002/000159 2000), CBD gave a positive effect in a maximal electroshock test, showed antinociceptive activity, *in vitro* inhibition of 5HT-induced contractions of guinea pig ileum, anti-inflammatory action in the rat paw oedema test (rat), antimicrobial activity (*in vitro*) and potentiation of hexabarbitone sleeping time. These pharmacological activities support the proposed use of a CBD-

TABLE 1. Comparison of Some Pharmacological Effects of THC and CBD

Effect	THC	CBD	Reference
CB1 (Brain receptors)	+ +	±	Pertwee et al., 1998
CB2 (Peripheral receptors)	+	−	
CNS Effects			
Anticonvulsant[†]	− −	+ +	Carlini et al., 1973
Muscle Relaxant	− −	+ +	Petro, 1980
Antinociceptive	+ +	+	
Catalepsy	+ +	+ +	
Psychotropic	+ +	−	
Antipsychotic	− −	+ +	Zuardi, 1997
Neuroprotective Antioxidant Activity*	+	+ +	Hampson A J et al., 1998
Antiemetic	+ +	−	
Sedation (reduced spontaneous activity)	+	+	Zuardi, 1997
Cardiovascular Effects			
Bradycardia	− −	+	Smiley et al., 1976
Tachycardia	+	−	
Hypertension[§]	+	−	
Hypotension[§]	−	+	Adams et al., 1977
Anti-inflammatory	±	±	Brown, 1998

* Effect is CB1 receptor independent.
† THC is pro convulsant.
§ THC has a biphasic effect on blood pressure; in naïve patients it may produce postural hypotension and it has also been reported to produce hypertension on prolonged usage.

rich cannabis extract in the treatment of severe arthritis (Burstein and Raz 1972).

QUALITY ISSUES

There is a compelling case for development of cannabis-based medicines using defined extracts as the active substance. GW Pharmaceuticals has developed a growing system that builds in quality by excluding the majority of adventitious factors, which normally have to be monitored and tolerated in field grown crops. Standardization and high quality have been achieved by growing specific chemovars under controlled conditions. However compelling the case for botanical extracts, it is essential that quality be built into the product. In order to do this it has been necessary to examine critically every aspect of the growing and production process. Field grown crops are subject to a range of factors adversely affecting quality. Recently, guidelines have been proposed for Good Agricultural Practice, expected to be incorporated into European Union (EU) legislation. These guidelines address many of the issues applicable to field grown crops. However, a more radical approach, giving an even higher degree of regulatory assurance, is to protect the plants from as many adventitious factors as possible by growing under glass in a controlled environment.

BOTANICAL SOURCE OF MEDICINAL CANNABIS

Hortapharm BV and GW Pharmaceuticals have produced a range of cannabis chemovars, which express a high proportion of their cannabinoid content as a specific chemical entity. This library contains chemovars that produce predominantly either THC, CBD, one of their precursors or congeners. This opens up the exciting prospect of using chemovars that produce some of the less well-studied cannabinoids such as tetrahydrocannabivarin (THCV) and cannabinodivarin (CBDV), which are characteristic of cannabis grown in South East Asia. The use of extracts from specific chemovars makes it possible to examine the effects of single extracts, or by blending extracts, to achieve a ratio of cannabinoids which may be optimal for a particular therapeutic condition. Initially, extracts from a high THC and a high CBD chemovar have been used to produce medicinal cannabis products. These contain predominantly THC, predominantly CBD or a defined ratio of THC and CBD.

The high THC chemovar is a stable hybrid of *Cannabis sativa*, subtype *indica* crossed with *Cannabis sativa*, subspecies *indica*. The principal cannabinoid produced (typically more than 94% of the total cannabinoid) is Δ^9-tetrahydrocannabinol with approximately 1.5% of cannabidiol.

The high CBD chemovar is a stable hybrid of *Cannabis sativa*, subtype *sativa* that has been heavily crossed and inbred with other varieties of *Cannabis sativa*. Typically, the principal cannabinoids produced in this chemovar have more than 90% of total cannabinoid as CBD, with approximately 3% present as THC. The exact details of the pedigree of these chemovars are the subject of Plant Breeders' Rights.

After selection for cannabinoid content, a group of chemovars is produced, but not all of them are equally hardy and suitable for volume production of cannabinoids. The plants are further selected for vigour and robustness. The production of standardized cannabis is from cuttings prepared from "mother" plants. This ensures that the genotype is fixed and there is consistency in the proportion of cannabinoids in each chemovar. Stability of cannabis biomass is also improved in these chemovars. Production quantities of cannabis are produced from seedless female plants.

Cannabis is a dioecious plant, and it is thus typical for male and female flowers to appear in separate plants. The male plant bears staminate flowers and the female plant carries pistillate flowers, which develop into the fruit and seeds. The content of useful cannabinoid is greatest in the flowering heads, particularly in the female plants. Monoecious plants may occur bearing both male and female flowers on different branches of the same plant. The appearance of male flowers results in early fertilization of female plants, with loss of yield. To optimize cannabinoid content it is essential to remove these "rogue" male flowers before they mature. Monoecious plants appear spontaneously in medicinal cannabis plants but are more frequent in varieties intensively bred for hemp production. In production of cannabis, the appearance of male flowers will result in fertilization of female plants, and reduction in yield of cannabinoids. For this reason plants bearing male flowers are removed as soon as they are detected. Raman (1998) has reviewed the process of masculinization of female plants in order to produce "self-varieties." Masculinization of female plants can be induced by chemical agents in order to produce self varieties for selective breeding (Ram and Sett 1982). A number of agents are known to induce masculinization including irradiation, treatment with streptovaricin and exposure to low levels of carbon monoxide.

Using a variety of techniques, De Meijer and Keizer (1996) have produced specific chemovars that have a very high content of total cannabinoids expressed as either THC or CBD. This programme of work has resulted in other chemovars that predominantly express cannabinoid content as specific cannabinoids other than THC and CBD.

In addition to fixation of the chemovars in terms of cannabinoid expression, it is necessary to further select for vigour. This has resulted in a series of chemovars that have the necessary robustness for large-scale production of cannabis in controlled conditions of lighting and temperature. This is the essence of the technology that has been developed by Hortapharm BV and GW Pharmaceuticals, after selection from accessions of material obtained from around the world.

The original (mother) plants are maintained in long day length to produce non-flowering, vegetative growth. The mother plants are used as a source of genetically identical cuttings (also referred to as clones). The clones are then grown on, and by manipulation of day length they are induced to flower and produce plants from which the product is prepared. A percentage of the young clone plants, when established, are retained under vegetative conditions (not allowed to flower) to produce further clones. The two chemovars used in the production of cannabis-based medicinal extract were selected from the range of varieties produced in this programme.

In the plant, cannabis resin is present in glandular trichomes. It is possible to obtain fractions containing a high concentration of resin by collecting these. Fractions rich in these trichomes constitute hashish, which may contain up to 60% of cannabis resin. However, for volume production it is more economic to harvest whole plants when the flowers are beginning to senesce, and to extract cannabinoids from the entire aerial parts of the plant.

HARVESTING

Field grown cannabis, if allowed to fall on the ground, is subject to fungal attack and contamination from birds and vermin. When grown on the small scale it is possible to hand pick the flowering tops from cannabis, but volume production demands mechanized means of harvesting and processing. When harvested, cannabis has moisture content of approximately 25%. In order to have a stable product it is necessary to reduce the moisture content to under 12%. Biomass stored away from light and heat is relatively stable. In the dried plant, a significant proportion of total cannabinoid is present as the cannabinoid acids (THCA and CBDA). These acids are not known to have cannabinergic activity and conversion of cannabinoid acids to free cannabinoids, the biologically active form, occurs spontaneously over time and is accelerated by heating. Smoking effectively decarboxylates cannabinoid acids. In other methods of preparation for medicinal use, it is necessary to ensure that this change is effected, as the cannabinoid acids do not have biological activity.

PREPARATION OF EXTRACTS

Historically, extracts of cannabis were prepared (BPC 1934) by percolation with 90% ethanol. Various galenical preparations have been used, including tinctures (ethanolic extracts). Solid extracts (solvent-free) have been used for preparation of finished dosage forms after the optional removal of solvent. The extract of cannabis is an oily resinous material, which is virtually insoluble in water.

Other solvents that have been used in an attempt to produce a purified extract of cannabis include fluorinated solvents such as heptafluropropane (HFA 227) and norflurane (HFA 134a). These solvents produce extracts that contain waxes and colouring agents, and a small amount of terpenes in addition to the cannabinoids.

A cleaner extract is produced by extraction with supercritical CO_2. In this process the majority of colouring matter and chlorophyll are left behind. The extract contains principally the cannabinoids but also some high molecular weight waxy ballast and sufficient terpenes to produce the characteristic scent of cannabis. Most of the ballast can be removed by chilling an alcoholic solution, a process referred to as "winterization." The winterized extract is an accessible material for production of liquid dosage forms using pharmaceutically acceptable solvent systems.

CHOICE OF DOSAGE FORM

Cannabis preparations have been administered by most routes commonly employed in the pharmaceutical industry. Historically, it was given in mixtures prepared from tinctures, and in the form of pills. In Victorian times plasters prepared from powdered drug were applied locally to relieve pain and with ointments represent the first attempts at transdermal application. Oily eye drops were also used for the treatment of glaucoma. Smoking is probably the fastest way of producing the pharmacological effects of cannabis in humans after intravenous injection. However effective as a mode of recreational use, smoking as a route of dosing for a prescription product can no longer be justified on ethical, medico-legal or safety grounds.

The sublingual route administration has shown a rate of absorption intermediate between that achieved by smoking and the oral (swallowed) route. Selection of a dose presentation based on extracts containing THC and CBD has produced a medicine that is organoleptically acceptable to the majority of patients. More importantly, the ability to take the medicine in small sub-doses has been invaluable in the investigation of efficacy and safety. The time course is such that the patient is able to take account of cognitive cues in timing the next dose increment. This allows patients to titrate the dose to a level where they achieve benefit and minimize unwanted side effects.

Recreationally, smoking is the commonest route of administration, closely followed by oral ingestion (brownies). Some patients with multiple sclerosis who smoke cannabis report relief of spasm and pain after the second or third puff of a cannabis cigarette. This implies very rapid transit to, and absorption into the central nervous system. The time involved is seconds rather than minutes. The oro-pharyngeal, buccal, sublingual and respiratory mucosae have venous drainage directly into the *vena cava* and the left side of the heart. Material absorbed through the mucosae of these areas is therefore not exposed to the liver during its first circuit into the systemic circulation. The drainage from the rest of the gastrointestinal tract (other than for the distal part of the rectal mucosae) perfuses the liver, the major detoxifying organ of the body. In addition to protecting the organism from ingested toxins, the liver also metabolizes medicaments, which are subject to the same chemical processes. Blood from the liver subsequently returns to the left side of the heart and reaches the rest of the systemic circulation. This first pass through the liver may result in the removal of a substantial proportion of an ingested medicament. In the case of cannabinoids, more than 95% of an ingested dose is metabolized during this first pass. This may contribute to the variability and timing to achieve maximal plasma concentration (C_{max}) and the time to achieve this maximum (T_{max}). In the case of cannabis there is a very wide variation in the values of C_{max} and T_{max} observed. A further complication is the rapid metabolism of tetrahydrocannabinol to 11-hydroxy-THC, which is also psychoactive. This occurs during the first pass through the liver and possibly through other tissues involved in the chain of absorption before cannabinoids reach the left side of the heart.

The areas of the respiratory/alimentary system having venous drainage into the systemic circulation, thus avoiding the first pass effect, are the mucous membrane of the buccal cavity, the sublingual area, the oro-pharynx, the respiratory tract, and the distal part of the rectum. The avoidance of the first pass effect is the rationale for the use of buccal, nasal, sublingual and suppository formulations. Each has advantages and disadvantages.

- Suppositories are subject to hygienic and patient compliance restriction.
- Formulations intended for administration to the nasal mucosae may cause pain or reflex sneezing, and in extreme cases cause irritation (Tashkin et al. 1973) and damage to the mucosae.
- Preparations intended for administration by inhalation have the advantage of speed of onset, but there is a direct irritant effect of THC *per se*, in addition to the irritant effect of the products of pyrolysis. Opinion is divided on the direct irritant effect of cannabinoids and it is possible that formulations that contain particles capable of being hydrated in their transit of the respiratory tract have lower irritancy.
- Sublingual formulations may stimulate the flow of saliva, and it is difficult for patients to avoid swallowing when substantial amounts of saliva are produced. If drugs applied to the sublingual mucosae are swallowed

the cannabinoids will be subject to the first pass effect and will therefore be less effective. This will result in proportionately higher levels of metabolic products.

- Buccal formulations where the product is held in contact with the parietal buccal membrane may be subject to the same limitations. Both sublingual and buccal formulations depend on the efficient transfer of medicament from a hydrophilic vehicle to the cell membrane of the sublingual or buccal mucosae. It is likely that absorption of cannabinoids takes place through the interstices in the membranes or by transfer into the epithelial cells. This transfer is governed principally by the lipid solubility of medicaments, and the partitioning of a lipid solid drug through an aqueous surface layer into a lipophilic absorption mechanism is an area for investigative research.

There are therefore a number of physical and biological limitations on the routes of administration of cannabinoids, but also opportunities for innovation in devising presentations to optimize administration. With the development of sensitive and specific methods of analysis, it is now possible to produce the kinetic profile that is best suited to treatment of specific therapeutic indications. Sublingual administration gives slower absorption than the respiratory route. However it is fast enough. The interval between doses allows time for subjects to become aware of the onset of cognitive changes in relation to wanted effects. Patients are thereby able to titrate doses to exploit the window between wanted therapeutic effects and unwanted side effects.

CLINICAL STUDIES

Initial phase 1 studies were carried out using a glycoalcoholic solution of cannabis extract, which was applied to the sublingual mucosae (Guy, Whittle and Grey 2000a and Whittle and Guy 2001). Fractional doses were given so that 2.5 mg was applied at intervals of 10 minutes.

The first human exposure to GW Pharmaceuticals (GWP) preparations of THC and CBD took place in healthy volunteers late in 1999. This placebo-controlled, six period, crossover study in six healthy volunteers assessed pharmacodynamic effects, pharmacokinetic profile, safety and tolerability including examination of routine clinical laboratory results and continuous monitoring of ECG and vital signs, cognitive effects, adverse events and subjective effects of a single dose of three cannabis based medicinal extracts (CBME) administered sublingually, and one formulation via aerosol and nebulizer.

CBME tested were High THC, High CBD, THC:CBD 1:1 mixture, and matching placebo. Maximum permitted dose was THC 20 mg and/or CBD 20 mg given incrementally at 10-minute intervals. All six subjects successfully completed the six periods of the study without giving rise to safety concerns. Pharmacokinetic profiles showed reliable absorption of CBME with peaks at 5 minutes following inhalation and approximately 2 h sublingually. Well-recognized effects of THC such as psychoactivity, conjunctival reddening, and intermittent tachycardia were observed. Overall, the cognitive effects were modest. Adverse effects reported by the subjects included vivid dreams, conjunctival injection, tachycardia, postural hypotension, hunger, pallor and sweating. No serious adverse effects were noted.

The design chosen by GWP for the initial clinical research is a series of double-blind, crossover, placebo-controlled single case studies. After an initial two week run-in period on open label THC:CBD 1:1 mixture, subjects enter a four way double blind crossover study comparing the 1:1 THC:CBD mixture, High THC, High CBD and placebo. After completion of this, patients are given the option of entering a long-term safety and tolerability follow-up study.

Sixty-four patients with a range of medical diagnoses including multiple sclerosis, spinal cord injury and other serious neurological conditions, have so far been titrated on to sublingual CBME. Of these, over 80% have chosen to continue receiving the medication in the long-term extensions. Between them, these subjects have now generated more than 950 patient-treatment weeks.

Virtually all the subjects remaining on treatment have experienced significant alleviation of at least one key symptom, and in some cases the improvement has been sufficient, in the patients own words, to transform lives by dramatically reducing pain. These improvements are particularly notable in that an inclusion criterion is intractability of symptoms in the face of available standard therapy. Among the positive effects recorded are relief of neuropathic pain, spasms, spasticity and bladder-related symptoms; at least partial alleviation of tremor; and improvements in mood and measures of overall well-being. Intoxication is the most frequent dose-limiting effect for the THC-containing medicines.

Because so little is known of optimal dose patterns for CBME, patients have been allowed to establish dose level and frequency by self-titration, with defined upper limits (no more than eight 2.5 mg doses within any 3 h period and no more than 120 mg/24 h). Many subjects chose to take small doses at more frequent intervals than the usual three or four times a day pattern. A wide range of individual daily dose requirements has been noted, but once a pattern is established very little variation within subject seems to occur. No evidence of tolerance to therapeutic effects has been noted so far. Most patients can achieve symptom relief at a sub-intoxication dose, although the margin between the two thresholds is often narrow.

A range of adverse effects has been reported, most of which seem to occur early in the treatment and diminish as a suitable dose is arrived at by self-titration. The most commonly occurring effects (i.e., those reported on 3 or more occasions) in descending order of frequency were headaches, nausea, burning in the mouth, intoxication, sweating, flu-like symptoms, vomiting, falls, and chest pain of unknown origin. Almost all of these effects have been transient, of only mild or moderate intensity, and well tolerated by the patients. One event defined as severe has been reported, but this ended in complete recovery following supportive treatment.

These pilot studies have provided important information which will inform future randomized, placebo-controlled cohort studies, including appropriate doses and dosing patterns, selection of CBME content for different conditions, identification of target symptoms and outcome measures. They have uncovered opportunities for optimization of the formulations (e.g., volume, solvents, taste, and blinding) and types of presentation, which can be incorporated into larger studies. With such small numbers, it is difficult to interpret the ultimate significance of adverse events. However, these preliminary studies have provided the investigators with invaluable hands-on experience of using cannabis-derived medicines in a therapeutic setting. They supplied further reassuring evidence of the safety and tolerability of these medicines in patients, often middle-aged or elderly, with serious medical disorders.

NON-SMOKING INHALATION

Non-smoking inhalation of cannabis is a fast and attractive route of administration for the new generation of cannabis-based medicines, which have been developed. The question arises, why not use smoking as a method of administration for a prescription product? The reasons are self-evident but are worth re-stating as this proposal periodically re-surfaces.

There are medico-legal implications involved in recommending smoking in any form. Cannabis, like other cellulosic materials, produces particulates and tar when burnt. These contain polyaromatic hydrocarbons (PAHs) known to be carcinogenic. The pattern of bronchial pre-carcinogenic cytological changes in habitual chronic cannabis smokers is similar to that of tobacco smokers. It is difficult to dissect out the contribution made by cannabis alone in this regard, since many cannabis smokers also smoke tobacco, and many study designs do not allow this variable to be assessed. Other factors that militate against the use of smoking as a route of administration for a prescription drug are the dislike of some patients for smoke and the perceived sociological disincentives expressed by some patients who do not wish to be seen smoking a street drug. Reports of an irritant effect of cannabis smoke are also a factor to be taken into account. Recreational smoking is a personal decision and is vigorously defended by users as a personal right. However, in the present climate of opposition to smoking in general, drug developers are unwilling to shoulder the moral and legal responsibility for adverse events resulting from recommending it as method of administration. There is, therefore, a search for non-smoking methods of administering cannabinoids via the respiratory tract. A number of methods of administration currently in use for other drugs have been examined for their applicability to administration of cannabinoids or extracts of cannabis.

The physical properties of medicaments given by inhalation are important. When air is inhaled through the nose it passes through the naso-pharynx and past the epiglottis into the trachea. The naso-pharynx acts as a filter to prevent the entry of large particles and has a role in warming (or cooling in the case of smoking) and humidifying the stream of air and particles. Air passing into the trachea enters the lung via the bronchi, bronchioles and alveoli. The bronchi walls contain rings of cartilage linked together with smooth muscle. Their inner surface is lined by cilia, which beat and assist the upward and outward movement of unwanted fine particles, which are then swallowed. The bronchioles are narrower versions of the bronchi, which do not have cartilage but are elastic; they constrict and dilate to modify the resistance to passage of air. Deeper within the lung the bronchioles branch repeatedly giving rise to terminal bronchioles, and the end outgrowths of the bronchioles are the alveoli. The walls of the respiratory bronchioles and alveoli are thin, covered in a network of fine capillaries and are the sites for gaseous and drug exchange. Products given by inhalation usually deliver the active ingredient in the form of aerosol droplets or as solid particles. In the case of cannabis, some of these particles may be condensed from vaporized cannabinoid that have subsequently become hydrated in the high relative humidity within the bronchial tree. The site at which droplets or particles are deposited in the lung depends largely on their aerodynamic diameter. This measure is the diameter of the perfect sphere that would fall through air at the same speed as the particle. Particles with an aerodynamic diameter greater than 10 micrometers tend to be deposited in the upper regions of the respiratory tract where they are quickly removed by the ciliated epithelium. Only particles approximately 2 micrometers or less are capable of reaching the alveoli. In the case of conventional drug particle inhalers, it is estimated that only 5-20% of the delivered dose reaches its site of action.

The relative humidity of the respiratory tract is approximately 99.5%, and inhaled particles, may hydrate and grow in size. Aerosolized liquid droplets may behave similarly. An equilibrium is attained with this type of particle when vapour pressure on the surface of the particle and in the respiratory tract are the same. This process may take only milliseconds to complete. Particles with an aerodynamic diameter of less than 1 micrometer may also be re-expired. Particles with a diameter of less than 0.5 micrometers display Brownian motion and a small fraction may be re-expired and lost. These factors are important in designing novel presentations of cannabis-based medicines for inhalational use.

The technology for producing aerosolized metered dose inhalers (MDIs) and drug-particle inhalers is well described, and attempts have been made to adapt this type of inhaler for delivery of cannabinoids. THC and CBD are virtually insoluble in physiological saline, but are soluble in high concentrations of ethanol. There are limits on the quantity of ethanol that can be taken into the respiratory tract. Vaporization of ethanol also produces both cooling and irritant effects. This greatly limits the amount of cannabinoid that can be administered per actuation of a pressurized device. Co-solvents such as propylene glycol and glycerol and surfactants produce marginal improvements in the concentration of cannabinoid, but a typical quantity that can be delivered (25-125 micro litres) using commercially available spray buttons is a trade off between solubility, volume and the irritant effect of the solvent.

VAPORIZERS

The challenge is to devise a vaporizer that produces the rapid effects of cannabis without the disadvantages of pyrolysed material and the consequent tar production. On the World Wide Web there are a number of sites where designs for vaporizers are posted. These consist of a source of heat, which is applied to a portion of cannabis herb, and a means for containing the volume of vapour, which is produced so that it can be inhaled in the stream of inspired air. Typically, the heat is applied in the form of an electrical heating element (soldering iron bit) or radiant heat from an incandescent light bulb. The fluidised bed principle has been applied in a device recently patented by Pate (1997). In this device a portion of cannabis herb is entrapped between two screens, and heated air is passed through the fluidised bed of cannabis and distills off the cannabinoids. The vapour so produced can then be inspired into the respiratory tract substantially free of particulates and smoke. Careful regulation of the temperature is necessary to ensure that distillation is carried out at a temperature below that at which cannabis pyrolyses.

Vaporizers, in which a concentrated extract of cannabis is heated to produce vapor, are under development. Electronic control of the energy applied to the heater ensures that the concentrated extract of cannabis is efficiently vaporized, without the production of pyrolysis products. The device generates the vapour during the course of a single inspiratory cycle in a manner intended to produce a profile of absorption in the patient similar to that obtained from a cannabis cigarette. The device is a portable self-contained unit, powered by rechargeable batteries and is controlled electronically. The control device has an algorithm which computes the energy required to produce vaporization in the dosage form, and switches current to effect vaporization at a temperature below that causing pyrolysis. The generation of vapour from the portion of medicament is done in the course of a single inspiration. The equipment also has provision for recording the date and time of use.

Control of and recording of the pattern of use are important from the standpoint of security. The recording of data on usage is an important factor in giving confidence to enforcement agencies, and monitoring of the supply by the pharmacist. The technology also provides an opportunity for data collection in the context of clinical trials monitoring and patient compliance. The method of secure dispensing and the device are the subject of UK and overseas patents (Guy, Whittle and Grey 2000b). The secure dispensing features of the equipment include a tamper-evident membrane, matching of the patient with prescription and a frangible linear link. This ensures that if the device is improperly used it locks up completely and cannot be operated. In addition to the recording and read-out of data relating to use, a simple and robust exchange scheme has been set up with pharmacist-supervised control of replacement and extension therapy.

NEBULIZERS

Nebulizers are in use for the administration of antimicrobial drugs, bronchodilators, corticosteroids and asthma treatments such as sodium chromoglycate. Nebulizers rely for their efficacy on provision of doses of medicament over a relatively prolonged period at correspondingly low concentration. A feature of nebulization is that the nebulisate is carried on a mist of water particles. Many types of nebulizer are in use, and a characteristic of the designs is that a fine mist of particles is generated in a flow of gas that is saturated with water vapour. This last feature facilitates breathing by ensuring that mucous is thinned and the epithelium of the respiratory tract does not dry out. Considerable ingenuity has been exercised in devising methods for generating a mist of particles. These include devices using a Venturi effect. Essentially, this consists of a jet of gas blowing across the end of a dip tube, the other end of which rests in a reservoir of liquid. The reduction in pressure draws water up the tube that is then converted into a spray. Smaller particles are separated from those with a high mass and kinetic energy, which are returned to the reservoir for recycling.

In the Halolite™ nebulizer, medicament solution is drawn up the central part of a rotating hollow-stemmed "T" bar, which throws off particles centripetally. Particles with a high mass hit the wall of the chamber, drain down into the reservoir and are recycled. Smaller particles are aspirated in the stream of inhaled air. This model of nebulizer has an algorithm that ensures that a portion of nebulisate is injected into the inspired air at a determined time. The amount of nebulisate retained within the respiratory tree by the use of this algorithm is in excess of 93%. Where the vehicle used contains volatile components it is necessary to make allowance for this as some fractionation may occur with variation in the amount of drug made available as nebulisate. The extent of lung deposition from different types of nebulizer is reviewed by Hardy, Newman and Knoch (1993).

Many commercial nebulizers are intended to provide a relatively low concentration of medicament, in a saturated atmosphere over a prolonged period of time. This is not the ideal for administration of cannabis. Smoked cannabis is rapidly effective and patients with MS report relief starting with the second or third draw. Davis, McDaniel et al. (1984), have described the complex changes occurring in a smoked marijuana cigarette. The amount of THC entering the respiratory system is probably in the range 5-10 mg of THC. An important characteristic of this type of administration is the pulsatile presentation of a discreet quantity of cannabinoid that allows the patient to discern cognitive effects following each draw. The patient can then regulate both the amount absorbed and rate of absorption. Patients with disabling pain claim that they can titrate the dose to obtain relief with the minimum unwanted cognitive effects.

The ability to achieve this window of therapeutic benefit without adverse events is also a difference between patients and recreational users. The object of non-smoking alternative methods of administration must be to mimic this pattern of delivery. A number of designs of nebulizer have been devised to increase the concentration of medicament in the nebulisate. Piezoelectric oscillators have been used to generate fine particles by forcing liquid through perforated plates into a stream of air or oxygen. This method of production results in a population of particles with a more uniform mass distribution. Ultrasonic energy can be used to produce a dense cloud of particles of uniform size, and there are proprietary devices based on this principle. A feature of this type of device is the rapid response made possible by switching electrical energy to the ultrasonic generator. This gives what is essentially a square wave function and the algorithm described in the secure dispensing patents (Guy, Whittle and Grey 2000b) can be used to control the rate and quantity of cannabinoid delivered during each respiratory cycle.

TRANSDERMAL ADMINISTRATION

Theoretically, the use of transdermal delivery systems for cannabinoids is attractive. The active constituents are lipid soluble, non-ionized, and of a molecular mass which is at the top end of the range normally considered feasible for transdermal absorption. However, in practice the results have to date been rather disappointing.

One traditional and spectacular way of collecting hashish reported by Samuelsson (1992) is for the operative to run through a crop of flowering cannabis and to allow resin to adhere to clothing and skin. Cannabis resin, which adheres easily to the body, is then scraped from the clothing and skin. Exposure of skin to resin containing high concentrations of cannabinoids has not been reported to produce intoxication. This would indicate that absorption of cannabinoids transdermally without further formulation is not extensive. Nevertheless, there are a number of patents that claim that significant plasma levels can be achieved by transdermal administration. This illustrates the contribution made by presentation and formulation.

To speed absorption, a number of systems have been designed to enhance transdermal delivery by energizing transport. These include:

• the use of ultrasonic stimulation of the skin
• iontophoresis
• incorporation of cannabinoids into liposomes, which are then incorporated into transdermal patches.

A function of skin is to protect the internal organs from the environment, and in the case of cannabis and cannabinoids it appears to do this well. The routes of entry through the skin are migration:

• through the epidermis
• into the dermis which is well served with capillaries
• diffusion into the interstitial cement surround cells
• diffusion into the lipophilic secretion in sebaceous glands and hair follicles.

Cannabinoids are very lipophilic. Although the principal cannabinoids are not ionized and have a molecular mass of around 300 and a high milligram potency, the transdermal flux is low in human skin. Touitou, Fabin, Danny and Almog (1988) compared permeation kinetic parameters through human and rat skin *in vitro*. Rat skin was found to be about 13 times more permeable to Δ^8-THC than human skin. Autoradiographs of horizontal sections showed that 24 hours after application the drug was concentrated in the *stratum corneum*, in the upper dermis and around hair follicles, indicating that THC penetrates the skin through lipophilic pathways. These studies also examined the effect of oleic acid as a permeation enhancer, and in rats a serum level of approximately 50 ng/ml of THC and metabolites (measured as cross-reacting cannabinoids) was maintained for about 24 hours.

Compensation for the lower transdermal flux in human skin can be made to some extent by increasing the effective area of the patch. However, a patch with an area of 50 cm^2 with a drug reservoir concentration of 26.5 mg/g was calculated to provide a blood concentration of 12 ng/ml for THC. A number of later patents, many of which are probably speculative, are based on reservoir, drug in matrix types of composition. Penetration enhancers include DMSO, azone and oleic acid, which are well-tried substances to produce this effect.

One factor, which does not appear to be addressed in patch patents, is the practical point of disposal. In order to achieve linear diffusion of any agent into the skin it is necessary to have a steep concentration gradient. This means that the patch must contain relatively large amounts of cannabinoids to ensure linearity of transfer through the skin initially, and the kinetics of absorption are such that the used patch may contain as much as 90-95% of the original dose. This presents a real problem of how the spent dosage unit is to be disposed. A spent patch is likely to contain sufficient cannabinoid for several doses by the oral route, or by smoking.

The formulation of cannabinoids for topical application to the skin in the form of liposomes has been proposed by Touitou (1996). The essential components of the liposomes are a phospholipid, a lower aliphatic alcohol (C2-4), with aqueous propylene glycol as the solvent. It is claimed that the hydro/alcoholic/glycolic phospholipid system increases the permeation rate of a range of active compounds including cannabinoids through the skin. Transdermal application produces an approximately constant plasma level of cannabinoids, but it remains to be seen whether the pharmacokinetic profile produced by such devices is clinically effective.

Current research into cannabinoids has revealed that the body possesses an endocannabinoid system. The system, which is present in nearly all phyla from *Hydra* upwards is characterized by cannabinergic mediators such as anandamide and 2-arachidonyl glycerol (2-AG) that are derived from substances quite different chemically from the plant cannabinoids. The analogy between cannabinoids, vanilloids and opioids is striking. In each case there is a plant material, which appears to bind to the same receptors as endogenous ligands. Research into novel cannabinergic compounds has followed a similar pattern to that employed in the case of opioids. It has polarized into a search for synthetic agonists, antagonists, reverse agonists or partial agonists using the paradigms familiar to the pharmaceutical industry in the development of analgesics to replace morphine. It is approximately 200 years since Setürner isolated morphine from opium and about 30 years since the discovery of different types of opioid receptors and the endorphins. The search for novel cannabinergic compounds should not take as long. In the meantime there is an alternative route to novel cannabis based medicines. It depends on a renewed search for novelty in the clinical application of cannabis extracts containing known combinations of cannabinoids. Not all of the actions of cannabis are based on receptors that are currently characterized, leaving open the possibility of further cannabinoid receptors. There are also other cannabinoids that have not been studied in the same detail as THC and CBD that may have clinical benefit.

In finding new cannabis-based medicines, an alternative to the pharmaceutical industry research approach is to build on the knowledge of receptor and non-receptor pharmacology and to explore the clinical benefit of these known compounds. It is probable that they will provide surprises in efficacy, but because man has already been exposed to them for thousands of years, they may not present so many problems in metabolism and toxicity.

REFERENCES

Adams, M.D., J.T. Earnhardt, B.R. Martin, L.S. Harris, W.L. Dewey, and R.K. Razdan. 1977. A cannabinoid with cardiovascular activity but no overt behavioral effects. *Experientia* 33:1204-1205.

Burstein, S. and A. Raz. 1972. Inhibition of prostaglandin E2 biosynthesis by D1-tetrahydrocannabinol. *Prostaglandins* 2:369-375.

Brown, D.T. 1998. *Cannabis: The genus Cannabis*. Amsterdam: Harwood Academic Publishers.

Carlini E.A., J.R. Leiter, M. Tannhauser, and A.C.Berardi. 1973. Cannabidiol and *Cannabis sativa* extract protect mice and rats against convulsive agents. *J Pharm Pharmacol* 25:664-665.

Davis, K.H., I.A. McDaniel, Jr., et al. 1984. Some smoking characteristics of marijuana cigarettes. In Stig, W.L. Dewey, R.E. Agurell. *The cannabinoids: Chemical, pharmacologic and therapeutic aspects*. San Diego, CA: Academic Press.

De Meijer, E.P.M., and L.C.P. Keizer. 1996. Patterns of diversity in *Cannabis. Genet Resourc Crop Evolut* 43:41-52.

Guy, G.W., B.A. Whittle and M.J. Grey. 2000a. Dose dispensing Apparatus. GB Pat Application 25809.5, Oct 20, 2000.

Guy, G.W., B.A. Whittle and M.J. Grey. 2000b. Secure dispensing of materials. GB Patent Application 25811.1, Oct 20, 2000.

Hampson, A.J., M. Grimaldi, J. Axelrod, and D. Wink. 1998. Cannabidiol and (−) 9-tetrahydrocannabinol are neuroprotective antioxidants. *Proc Nat Acad Sci* 95: 8268-8273.

Hardy, J.G., S.P. Newman, and M. Knoch. 1993. Lung deposition from four nebulizers. *Resp Med* 87: 461-465.

House of Lords Science and Technology Sub Committee report. 2001. The development of prescription cannabis-based medicines (Jan 2001).

In-house Report GPA 002/000159. 2000. CBD Primary Screening Program.

Iversen, L.L. 2000. *The science of marijuana*. Oxford: Oxford University Press.

Mechoulam, R. (ed.) 1976. *Cannabinoids as therapeutic agents*. Boca Raton, FL: CRC Press.

Merck index: An encyclopedia of chemicals, drugs, and biologicals. 1996. S. Budavari, and M.J. O'Neil (Eds.), 12th Edition, Boca Raton, FL: CRC Press.

Merck's manual. 1899. Part 1, p. 26.

Pate, D. 1997. US Patent Application Number 08/919317, 28 August 1997.

Pertwee, R.G. 1998. Advances in cannabinoid receptor pharmacology in cannabis. pp. 125-174, in D.T. Brown (Ed.). *Cannabis: The genus Cannabis.* Amsterdam: Harwood Academic Publishers.

Petro, D.J. 1980. Marijuana as a therapeutic agent for muscle spasm or spasticity. *Psychosom* 21(1):81-85.

Price, M.A.P., and W.G. Notcutt. 1998. Cannabis in pain relief. pp. 223-246. In D.T. Brown (Ed.). *Cannabis: The genus Cannabis.* Amsterdam: Harwood Academic Publishers.

Raman, A. 1998. The cannabis plant: Botany, cultivation and processing for use. pp. 29-54. In D.T. Brown (Ed.). *Cannabis: The genus Cannabis.* Amsterdam: Harwood Publishers.

Ram, H.Y.M., and R. Sett. 1982. Reversal of ethephon-induced feminization in male plants of cannabis by ethylene antagonists. *Zeitschrift fur pflanzenphysiologie* 107(1):85-89.

Samuelsson, G. 1992. *Drugs of natural origin.* Stockholm, Sweden: Swedish Pharmaceutical Press.

Smiley, K.A., R. Karber, and S.A. Turkanis. 1976. Effect of cannabinoids on the perfused rat heart. *Res Comm Chem Pathol Pharmacol* 14:659-675.

Tashkin, D.P., B.J. Shapiro, and I.M. Frank. 1973. Acute pulmonary and physiological effects of smoked marijuana and oral delta-9-THC in healthy young men. *N Eng J Med* 289(7):336-341.

Touitou, E. 1996. US Patent 5,540,934 (July 30, 1996).

Touitou, E., B. Fabin, S. Danny, and S. Almog. 1988. Transdermal delivery of tetrahydrocannabinol. *Int J Pharmaceut* 43:9-15.

Whittle, B.A., and G.W. Guy. 2001. Formulations for sublingual delivery. GB Patent Application 103638.3, Feb 14, 2001.

Zuardi, A.W., and F.S. Guimarães. 1997. Cannabidiol as an anxiolytic and antipsychotic. In M.L. Mathre (Ed.), *Cannabis in medical practice.* Jefferson, NC and London: McFarland & Co. pp. 133-141.

Index

monoterpenes-related detoxification
of, 112,114
Δ^3-Carene, 114,119
Carvacrol, 114-115
α-Caryophyllene, 113,118
β-Caryophyllene, 112,115
CBC. *See* Cannabichromene
CBD. *See* Cannabidiol
CBG. *See* Cannabigerol
CBN. *See* Cannabinol
CD4+-CD8+ T-lymphocytes ratio,
effect of terpenoids on, 116
CD4+T lymphocytes
effect of cannabis on, 77
effect of dronabinol on, 77
as HIV infection marker, 6,7
effect of Δ^9-THC on, 65
Ceftriaxone, 64
Cell differentiation, effect of
cannabinoid receptors on, 73
Cell-mediated immunity, effect of
Δ^9-THC on, 62,66
Central nervous system, cannabis
smoke absorption by,
193-194
Central nervous system activity, of
inhaled cannabis compounds,
122
Cerebroprotective properties, of
cannabinoids, 68
c-Fos protein, 107
Chemokines, effect of cannabinoids
on, 65-66
Chemotherapy patients, Δ^9-THC-
related antiemesis in, 7-8
Chemovars, of cannabis, 184
as source of therapeutic extracts,
190-192
Chest pain, cannabis extracts-related,
197
Children, chemotherapy-related
antiemesis treatment in,
108-109

Cholesterol synthesis,
monoterpenes-related
inhibition of, 112,114
Christian Coalition, 19
Chronic obstructive pulmonary disease
correlation with cannabis smoking,
90,137-138
tobacco smoking-related, 90
1,8-Cineole, 113,117-118
Citronellol, 115,116
c-Jun protein, 107
Clinical trials
of AIDS treatments, 19
of cannabis
as an antiemetic, 8
government approval of, 31-32
government opposition to, 27-31
in United Kingdom, 185
of cannabis extracts, 195-197
Clinton Administration, 29,31
Clones, 192
Clostridium perfringens,
monoterpenoid-related
inhibition of, 118
CNN (television news network), 27
Cocaine, 76-77
Codeine
long-term use of, lack of tolerance
development in, 173
opium content of, 147
Cognex®, 117
Colon cancer, limonene prophylaxis
against, 116
Combustion, of cannabis, 122
Compassionate Use Investigational
New Drug Program,
17,21,23,24
termination of, 24,26-27
Consciousness, effect of cannabis on,
48-49
Constantine, Thomas, 31
Constipation, opium-related, 147
Controlled Substance Analogue
Enforcement Act of 1986,
109

Printed in the United States
by Baker & Taylor Publisher Services